APHASIOLOGY

Volume 22   Number 11   November 2008

CONTENTS

APHASIOLOGY

SUBSCRIPTION INFORMATION

Subscription rates to Volume 22, 2008 (12 issues) are as follows:
To institutions (full subscription): £1,263.00 (UK);   €1,668.00 (Europe); $2,085.00 (Rest of the world).
To institutions (online only):   £1,199.00 (UK);   €1,584.00 (Europe); $1,980.00 (Rest of the world).
An Institutional subscription to the print edition also includes free access to the online edition for any number of concurrent users across a local area network.
Subscriptions purchased at the personal (print only) rate are strictly for personal, non-commercial use only. The reselling of personal subscriptions is strictly prohibited. Personal subcriptions must be purchased with a personal cheque or credit card. Proof of personal status may be requested. For full information please visit the Journal's homepage.
To individuals: £531.00 (UK);   €702.00 (Europe); $878.00 (Rest of the world).
A subscription to the print edition includes free access for any number of concurrent users across a local area network to the online edition. ISSN 1464-5041.
Print subscriptions are also available to individual members of the British Aphasiology Society (BAS), on application to the Society.
Aphasiology now offers an iOpenAccess option for authors. For more information, see: www.tandf.co.uk/journals/iopenaccess.asp

For a complete and up-to-date guide to Taylor & Francis's journals and books publishing programmes, visit the Taylor and Francis website: http://www.tandf.co.uk/

Aphasiology (USPS 001413) is published monthly by Psychology Press, 27 Church Road, Hove, BN3 2FA, UK. The 2008 US Institutional subscription price is $2085.00. Periodicals Postage Paid at Jamaica, NY 11431, by US Mailing Agent Air Business Ltd, c/o Worldnet Shipping USA Inc., 149-35 177th Street, Jamaica, New York, NY 11434, USA. US Postmaster: Send address changes to *Aphasiology* (PAPH), Air Business Ltd, C/O Worldnet Shipping USA Inc., 149-35 177th Street, Jamaica, New York, NY 11434, USA.
Dollar rates apply to subscribers in all countries except the UK and the Republic of Ireland where the pound sterling price applies. All subscriptions are payable in advance and all rates include postage. Journals are sent by air to the USA, Canada, Mexico, India, Japan and Australasia. Subscriptions are entered on an annual basis, i.e., from January to December. Payment may be made by sterling cheque, dollar cheque, international money order, National Giro, or credit card (AMEX, VISA, Mastercard).

Orders originating in the following territories should be sent direct to the local distributor.
India: Universal Subscription Agency Pvt. Ltd, 101-102 Community Centre, Malviya Nagar Extn, Post Bag No. 8, Saket, New Delhi 110017.
Japan: Kinokuniya Company Ltd, Journal Department, PO Box 55, Chitose, Tokyo 156.
USA, Canada and Mexico: Psychology Press, a member of Taylor & Francis, 325 Chestnut St, Philadelphia, PA 19106, USA
UK and other territories: Psychology Press, c/o T&F Customer Services, Informa UK Ltd, Sheepen Place, Colchester, Essex, CO3 3LP, Tel: +44 (0)20 7017 5544; Fax: +44 (0)20 7017 5198; UK. E-mail: tf.enquiries@tfinforma.com

Typeset by H. Charlesworth & Co. Ltd., Wakefield, UK, and printed by Hobbs the Printers Ltd., Totton, Hants, UK. The online edition can be reached via the journal's website: http://www.psypress.com/aphasiology

Back issues: Taylor & Francis retains a three-year back issue stock of journals. Older volumes are held by our official stockists: Periodicals Service Company, 11 Main Street, Germantown, NY 12526, USA, to whom all orders and enquiries should be addressed. Tel: +1 518 537 4700; Fax: +1 518 537 5899;
E-mail: psc@periodicals.com; URL: http://www.periodicals.com/tandf.html

APHASIOLOGY, 2008, 22 (11), 1123–1126

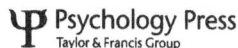

Editorial

Wolfram Ziegler and Ingrid Aichert

City Hospital Bogenhausen, München, Germany

We speak in syllables, not in phonemes or words. This idea, which dates back to Crompton (1982) and was revived in a series of experiments by Levelt and Wheeldon (1994), has been most influential in speech research during the last decade. The concept of a "mental syllabary", i.e., a store of syllable-sized motor planning units, has become a cornerstone in the modelling of spoken language production (Levelt, Roelofs, & Meyer, 1999).

One of the basic arguments in favour of the syllable as a core unit of articulation is based on the observation that a relatively small number of syllables occur very frequently, i.e., are articulated exceedingly often by the speakers of a language, and have thereby acquired the status of a highly overlearned, automated motor pattern. As an example, the German syllable [man] occurs 4082 times in a million words (CELEX; Baayen, Piepenbrock, & Gulikers, 1995). If it is true that we produce, on the average, more than 15,000 words each day (Mehl, Vazire, Ramírez-Esparza, Slatcher, & Pennebaker, 2007), and if we estimate that the average syllable number of German word tokens is 1.9 (CELEX count), we can infer that a German speaker's articulatory muscles are orchestrated to produce [man] approximately 116 times per day and more than 40,000 times every year. Such extensive motor exercise entails that over the years of speech acquisition the ensemble of gestures representing the syllable [man] acquires some kind of hard-wired representation, enabling us to access the whole motor pattern with high speed and high accuracy, and with only few attentional resources.

How then do we produce syllables that are not stored as ready-made motor programs? The German syllable [mɔk], for example, has a CELEX frequency of only 4 per million, hence its motor pattern is not exercised to any significant extent (approximately 20 times per year) and therefore probably does not make it into the mental syllabary. Nonetheless, everyday experience tells us that an adult speaker who encounters [mɔk] in a word by no means performs like a 2-year-old language learner; i.e., struggles for its pronunciation or simplifies it to something like [gɔk] or [mɔm]. Instead, no apparent difference is heard between frequent and infrequent syllables in everyday conversations of adult speakers, meaning that we must dispose of some very powerful alternative route of phonetic encoding, one that assembles the gestures for words and phrases from units smaller than the syllable. Levelt's model offers such an "indirect route" option of phonetic encoding (Levelt et al., 1999).

© 2008 Psychology Press, an imprint of the Taylor & Francis Group, an Informa business
http://www.psypress.com/aphasiology   DOI: 10.1080/02687030701820360

Given that there is still a vast difference between adult productions of new or infrequent syllables on the one hand, and a child's early attempts at speaking on the other, an indirect assembly route of adult speech must be based on extensively overlearned patterns as well. However, we still have little knowledge about which sub-syllabic routines we have learned during the long period of acquiring this formidable skill: Is it something like a universal set of gestural level coordinative structures? Is it an inventory of phonemes, of syllable onsets/rimes, or of bi-phonemes? Or is it a hierarchical motor network interleaving several representational levels? Moreover, if it is true that we dispose of precompiled syllabic motor programs and sub-syllabic routines at the same time, how are these two levels of motor representations related with each other? Are syllabic motor programs opaque, holistic units, or do they perhaps carry the imprints of the architecture of our sub-syllabic speech motor skills? And, furthermore, is the syllable really the highest structure of overlearned phonetic encoding processes? Or do we not also dispose of *rhythmic* skills, embracing two or more syllables, which must be considered part of the automated motor routines used in speaking?

Despite all these open questions, the idea of a deposit where ready-made, syllable-sized motor programs for speaking are stored has proved extraordinarily fertile in the field of *neuro*linguistics. There is significant interest in the syndrome of apraxia of speech, since this disorder is considered to interfere with the phonetic encoding stage of speaking (Code, 1998), and therefore qualifies as a hotspot for discussions concerning the architecture of phonetic representations. Volume 15 of *Aphasiology*, published in 2001, provided a platform for a lively debate of this issue, with a target article by Varley and Whiteside postulating that apraxic speakers have lost access to the syllabary and are cut down on the utilisation of an indirect encoding route (Varley & Whiteside, 2001). The discussion is still going on, and empirical data countering the "dual-route" hypothesis have been published ever since.

Beyond apraxia of speech, however, the notion of syllable frequency and the question of the significance of syllabic representations has conquered other fields of neurolinguistic inquiry as well, e.g., phonemic paraphasia, neologistic jargon, aphasic recurring utterances, dyslexia, language of demented people, or develop-mental speech impairment.

This special issue of *Aphasiology* presents a cross-section of the current discussion on the role of the syllable in speech and language processing in neurologic and neurodegenerative disorders. The idea of composing such an overview emerged on an informal meeting initiated by Ingrid Aichert, Prisca Stenneken, and Marina Laganaro,[1] and some of the contributions presented at this meeting are included on the pages to follow.

Cholin opens with an up-to-date overview of the role of the mental syllabary in speech production, trying to reconcile old and new psycholinguistic data with recent evidence from clinical studies. Stenneken, Hofmann, and Jacobs follow with a comparison of the sublexical properties of neologistic utterances of a Wernicke's aphasic patient with statistical properties of standard German, concluding that the impairment underlying phonemic jargon is constrained by structural properties of the syllable. In a third article, Janßen and Domahs then "go on with optimised feet", discussing the syllable at the crossroads of segmental and metrical structure. They

---

[1] *The Syllable and Beyond: Evidence from Disordered Speech.* Munich, 1 April 2006.

present data from a patient with a primary progressive aphasia who was remarkable for her pattern of segmental and metrical errors in reading and repetition. The paper contributed by Carreiras, Baquero, and Rodríguez draws on the observation that visual word recognition in transparent orthographies like Spanish is to a large extent affected by properties of the syllabic constituents of a word. They utilise this evidence to investigate if such syllable effects are observable in patients with Alzheimer's disease. Their findings suggest that the structural processing of written words at the syllabic level is preserved in this population, whereas the inhibitory processes released by syllable representations are impaired.

The last four contributions to this special issue of *Aphasiology* are devoted to the role of the syllable in apraxia of speech. Laganaro's article reports syllable frequency effects on speech errors in three individuals with apraxia of speech and brings up the riddle that a similar effect was also observable in three patients with conduction aphasia. How come? She presents a tentative explanation. A further confirmation of syllable frequency and syllable structure effects on accuracy of articulation in apraxia of speech is presented in Staiger and Ziegler's article. This contribution reports data from large samples of spontaneous speech and contributes to the question of whether, in conversational speech, apraxic speakers use words whose sublexical properties are statistically comparable to normal spontaneous speech, or if they avoid difficult things. Aichert and Ziegler tackle the problem of the holistic nature of syllabic representations by a learning experiment with apraxic speakers. They report on generalisation effects from the learning of simple CVC-syllables to more complex expansions of such forms, suggesting that syllable-sized motor programs are not structurally opaque, but have an internal organisation. The last paper by Ziegler, Thelen, Staiger, and Liepold concludes with a model-based analysis of apraxic speech errors in a word repetition task. The authors of this article end with the hypothesis that phonetic encoding spans several layers of word form representations.

Altogether we have collected a variegated bouquet of new data on and around the syllable in disordered speech and language. We are grateful to the authors in this special issue of *Aphasiology* for their valuable contributions and also for their help in cross-reviewing all the articles. We would also like to thank the external reviewers whose comments were extraordinarily helpful and who finally contributed a lot to the success of this endeavour. Last but not least, our thanks go to Chris Code, who was open-minded enough to invite us to take on some editorial duties and guest edit this collection of articles.

REFERENCES

Baayen, R. H., Piepenbrock, R., & Gulikers, L. (1995). *The CELEX lexical database*. [CD-ROM]. Linguistic Data Consortium, University of Pennsylvania, Philadelphia.

Cholin, J., Levelt, W. J. M., & Schiller, N. O. (2006). Effects of syllable frequency in speech production. *Cognition, 99*, 205–235.

Code, C. (1998). Major review: Models, theories and heuristics in apraxia of speech. *Clinical Linguistics and Phonetics, 12*, 47–65.

Crompton, A. (1982). Syllables and segments in speech production. In A. Cutler (Ed.), *Slips of the tongue and language production* (pp. 109–162). Amsterdam: Mouton Publishers.

Levelt, W. J. M., Roelofs, A., & Meyer, A. S. (1999). A theory of lexical access in speech production. *Behavioral and Brain Sciences, 22*, 1–75.

Levelt, W. J. M., & Wheeldon, L. R. (1994). Do speakers have access to a mental syllabary? *Cognition, 50*, 239–269.

Mehl, M. R., Vazire, S., Ramírez-Esparza, N., Slatcher, R. B., & Pennebaker, J. W. (2007). Are women really more talkative than men? *Science, 317*, 82.

Varley, R., & Whiteside, S. (2001). What is the underlying impairment in acquired apraxia of speech. *Aphasiology, 15*, 39–49.

APHASIOLOGY, 2008, 22 (11), 1127–1141

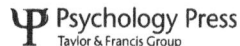

The mental syllabary in speech production: An integration of different approaches and domains

Joana Cholin

Johns Hopkins University, Baltimore, MD, USA

Background: The assumption of independently stored syllable motor programs has become an inherent part of the speech production model by Levelt and colleagues (Levelt, 1989, 1992; Levelt, Roelofs, & Meyer, 1999; Levelt & Wheeldon, 1994). In this model a mental syllabary is assumed to be located between the levels of phonological and phonetic encoding and is thought to contain the (high-frequency) syllables of a given language as ready-made whole gestural scores. The retrieval of precompiled syllable programs allows for rapid and fluent articulation and reduces the computational load relative to a segment-by-segment online assembly. A second online assembly is assumed to generate syllable programs for low-frequency and new syllables.

Aims: The aim of the current paper is to analyse and compare the findings from two different lines of research that investigated the notion of a mental syllabary in speech production: psycholinguistic studies on the one hand and clinical studies on the other hand. Both lines of research rest on the assumption that high- and low-frequency syllables involve different retrieval or assembly mechanisms: If high-frequency syllables are stored and can be retrieved as whole entities, retrieval times should both be faster and more accurate compared to low-frequency syllables that need to be assembled.

Main Contribution: The joint analysis of these two lines of research might reveal insights into the underlying mechanisms of phonological/phonetic encoding. Whereas there seems to be converging evidence for the assumption that high-frequency syllables are stored, the mechanisms that generate low-frequency syllables are less clear.

Conclusion: Taken altogether, the emerging picture shows that further research is needed in order to fully understand how the mental syllabary and related representations and processes interact. The integration of results from the two different domains, psycholinguistics and clinical research, might offer means for a deeper understanding, helping to further specify the mental syllabary theory.

Keywords: Speech production; Word-form encoding; Mental syllabary; Syllable-frequency effects.

A SKETCH OF THE MENTAL SYLLABARY

The fluency and speed of overt speech requires the spatial and temporal coordination of consecutive articulatory units that form connected speech. If we think of connected speech as a string composed of a small set of beats, representing a basic articulatory unit, which recur time and again, then the fundamental idea of

Address correspondence to: Joana Cholin, Johns Hopkins University, Department of Cognitive Science, 237 Krieger Hall, 3400 N. Charles Street, Baltimore, MD 21218, USA. E-mail: jocholin@cogsci.jhu.edu

The author wishes to thank Karen Croot, Wolfram Ziegler, Ingrid Aichert, Ansgar Hantsch, Alissa Melinger, and Jeremiah W. Bertz for helpful comments on earlier versions of this manuscript.

 DOI: 10.1080/02687030701820352

pre-compiled and stored motor programs that facilitate the fluency of spoken language is best understood. Indeed, a relatively small number of beats, or syllables, comprise most of our daily spoken production. However, spoken language production is by no means a simple concatenation of isolated motor programs— on the contrary, it is very difficult to identify discrete units in the continuous acoustic output, which unfolds incrementally over time without clear pauses, boundaries, or delimitation. Due to various phonological/phonetic processes, such as allophonic variation, coarticulation, and (the resulting) assimilation, a given articulatory unit is not completely determined by its underlying (abstract) motor program. The realisation of the same syllable, uttered in isolation or in identical contexts, will always be slightly different, but it is nevertheless the same syllable. It is the unchanging and recurring core of a syllable (independent of the environments in which this syllable may appear) that is hypothesised to be stored as an abstract motor program in the syllabary. Thus, these stored motor programs are *abstract* in the sense that they can flexibly be adjusted to various rapidly changing phonological/ phonetic environments. At the same time, they are *concrete* enough that the storage of this motor program is highly efficient for the cognitive system relative to the computational load of a segment-by-segment online-assembly of the same motor program. Crucially, the syllable motor programs in the syllabary do in some sense already incorporate some context dependencies of (also recurring) environments.

In the Levelt, Roelofs, and Meyer (1999) model of speech production, which explicitly incorporates the mental syllabary, syllabification is an online process that takes place relatively late during word form encoding, namely after the word forms have been retrieved from long-term memory. According to the Levelt et al. model, the phonemes in the stored word forms are not specified for internal syllabic position such as onset or coda. This is a critical assumption in the Levelt et al. model and contrasts with other models of language production which assume that word forms are specified for syllable positions (in particular Dell, 1986, 1988; see also Costa & Sebastián-Gallés, 1998, and Sevald, Dell, & Cole, 1995). The main argument for not pre-determining syllabic positions in the stored word forms derives from the phenomenon of *resyllabification*. In connected speech, syllable boundaries often differ from a word's or morpheme's canonical syllabification due to morphopho- nological processes such as inflection, derivation or cliticisation (Booij, 1995). The ubiquity of such resyllabifications in spoken speech production renders pre- specification of segments to syllable positions highly inefficient (e.g., Schiller, Meyer, Baayen, & Levelt, 1996). The domain of syllabification is the phonological word, which can be smaller or larger than the lexical word. If, for instance, the stored phonological code for the word *defend* is syllabified (i.e., as de.fend),[1] then the speaker must "resyllabify" the word when used in a different context, such as the different inflectional forms like the past tense (de.fen.ded) or cliticisation (defend it– de.fen.dit). Accordingly, the phonemes that were spelled out from memory are incrementally bundled together, proceeding from left to right, to form syllable-sized abstract phonological packages. The syllables "did" and "dit" constitute high- frequency syllables in English that emerge after the corresponding morphemes have been retrieved from memory and syllabified conjointly during phonological encoding. This "bundling" follows language-specific syllabification rules as well as

---

[1] A dot indicates a syllable boundary.

universal syllabification constraints such as maximisation of onsets and sonority gradations. Thus, syllabification is a vastly context-dependent process that flexibly generates abstract phonological syllables in recurring phonological environments.

As soon as an abstract phonological syllable is generated, further phonetic encoding can take place. Potentially, there are two mechanisms or routes that can be engaged to transform an abstract phonological syllable into a phonetic syllable that will prepare the ground for articulation. One route, often called the *direct* route, involves the retrieval of motor programs for syllables or *gestural scores* from the hypothesised syllabary. The term *"gesture"* or *"gestural score"* refers to a notion in *articulatory phonology* (Browman & Goldstein, 1992) in which discrete (constricting) actions of distinct organs or articulators, the so-called gestures, form the basic phonological units. In that sense, the stored syllables within the syllabary are combinations of different gestural scores or atoms of constricting gestures. The assumption of whole gestural scores for syllables adopts the idea that stored syllables' motor programs are abstract representations of the gestures that have to be performed at different articulatory tiers: a glottal tier, a nasal tier, and an oral tier. The actual details of the movements in realising the scores, such as lip protrusion and jaw lowering, are within the domain of the articulatory system (Goldstein & Fowler, 2003). According to Levelt (1989), stored syllables can be pronounced with more or less force, with shorter or longer duration, and with different kinds of pitch movements. These are free parameters, which have to be set from case to case.

Accessing the mental syllabary and activation of syllable motor programs in the syllabary is assumed to follow the same criteria that are described for lemma selection from the mental lexicon (Levelt, 2001; Roelofs, 1997a, 1997b; 2002a, 2002b). The activation of syllables is simulated in WEAVER++ (Word-Encoding by Activation and VERification) which is the spreading activation based network model developed by Roelofs (1992, 1997a, 1997b, 1999, 2002b) that is based on Levelt's (1989, 1992) and Levelt et al.'s (1999) theory of speech production. In WEAVER++, each segment that partakes in the phonological syllables spreads activation to all other syllable programs that also contain these segments. In this way, numerous syllables receive activation. When one of the (co)activated syllables exceeds threshold, a production rule verifies the link between the segments of the syllable in the syllabary and the phonological syllable that was incrementally composed one level up. When the target syllable node has been selected, further phonetic fine tuning will adjust the consecutive syllables.

The *indirect* route of phonetic encoding has been proposed for the construction of new or very low-frequency syllables. The evidence for the notion of a qualitatively different route operating in phonetic encoding is limited but it cannot be disputed that there must be a mechanism that constructs phonetic syllables from scratch. How would we otherwise imagine that infants form syllabic patterns or adults acquire syllables of a foreign language or produce novel syllables? Accordingly, there must be an alternative online segment-by-segment assembly mechanism to transform phonological syllables into phonetic syllables. This route could operate outside, i.e., alongside, the syllabary or within the syllabary by combining smaller units (such as demisyllables or onsets and rhymes) to create motor programs that are not stored as such.

If there is in fact an alternative route which might be less automatic than the retrieval route via the syllabary, it cannot be excluded that this route can also be used for the assembly of high-frequency syllables; for instance, in cases when more conscious on-line control of speech production is required. If there are in fact two distinct mechanisms, i.e., an online assembly operation alongside the syllabary, then the question arises of whether or not these two routes are always active, i.e., run in parallel. Crucially, the retrieval of ready-made motor programs that are stored as whole units should be faster and less error prone. The questions of how potentially different routes of phonetic encoding operate and how they possibly interact remain open, and it can only be speculated how the frequency of a syllable determines which route will be used in changing contexts (see also Miller, 2001). The issue of an additional process that operates on subsyllabic units or even single phonemes is critical and will be discussed in more detail throughout the present article.

The final step in speech planning involves the articulatory network, a coordinative motor system that includes feedback mechanisms (Goldstein & Fowler, 2003; Saltzman, 1986, Saltzman & Kelso, 1987) that transforms these articulatory plans into overt speech.

STORED SYLLABIC MOTOR PROGRAMS

The usefulness of storing frequent syllables was underscored in an analysis by Schiller and colleagues (Schiller, Meyer, Baayen, & Levelt, 1996) which demonstrated that 80% of all speech in languages such as English, Dutch, and German can be produced with the 500 most frequent syllables, even though these languages consist of more than 12,000 syllables in total. Thus, the tens of thousands of words in any given language are composed of a relatively small inventory of syllables. This parsimony assumption, that the storage of highly overused motor programs is very efficient cognitively, is not restricted to language and is in line with studies investigating other types of stored motor units, e.g., stored hand movements (Buxbaum & Coslett, 2001; Buxbaum, Kyle, & Menon, 2005). Thus, the stable and unchanging parts of articulatory programs are stored in long-term memory (possibly in a repository in a pre-motor area; Dronkers, 1996; Indefrey & Levelt, 2000; Kerzel & Bekkering, 2000), composed of specific combinations of segments organised in(to) one syllable (possibly in a hierarchical manner, see Aichert & Ziegler, 2008 this issue; Ziegler, Thelen, Staiger, & Liepold, 2008 this issue). The finding that many of the coarticulatory properties of a word are syllable-internal—that is, that there is more gestural dependence within a word's syllables than between its syllables (Browman & Goldstein 1988; Byrd 1995, 1996)[2]—underpins the assumption of stored whole-gestural scores for entire syllables, as opposed to larger units such as words or smaller units such as single segments.

Direct and indirect evidence for stored syllables stems from a variety of studies using different experimental paradigms: syllable-priming studies, implicit priming studies, and (most importantly) syllable frequency studies. In nearly a dozen syllable-priming studies carried out in different languages, researchers tried to prime the first syllable of disyllabic target words by presenting a visual syllable prime that was identical to the initial syllable of the to-be-named target word (Dutch: Baumann, 1995; Schiller, 1998; Schiller, Meyer, & Levelt, 1997; Mandarin Chinese: Chen, Lin, & Ferrand, 2003; French: Brand, Rey, & Peereman, 2003; Evinck, 1997; Ferrand, Segui, & Grainger, 1996; Schiller, Costa, & Colomé, 2002; English: Ferrand, Segui, & Humphreys, 1997; Schiller, 1999, 2000; Schiller & Costa, 2006; for Spanish and an

---

[2] Coarticulatory effects that cross syllable boundaries (as discussed, e.g., by Farnetani 1990; Recasens 1984, 1987) are ascribed to the motor execution system.

overview see Schiller et al., 2002). In all these studies, a syllabic prime was given which was either congruent with the target's syllabic structure (e.g., *ba* as a prime for *ba*.sis or *bas* as a prime for *bas*.ket) or incongruent (e.g., *ba* as a prime for *bas*.ket or *bas* as a prime for *ba*.sis). The majority of these studies found a segmental overlap effect rather than a syllable-priming effect; i.e., phonologically related primes, independent of their syllabic relation to the target word, facilitated the response relative to unrelated control primes, with longer CVC primes being more effective than CV primes (for more details see Schiller, 2004). The failure to detect a syllable-priming effect with this task has been explained by the fact that the priming method taps into higher-level processes related to phonological encoding but does not access later stages of syllable retrieval. Subsequently, versions of the *implicit* priming method (Meyer, 1990, 1991) were used to trace the emergence of syllables at later stages of word form encoding. Using a modified version of the *implicit priming paradigm*, Cholin, Schiller, and Levelt (2004) found preparation effects for syllables that were implicitly given prior to disyllabic target words that had to be produced. Together with the unsuccessful syllable-priming studies that failed to identify syllabic units at higher levels, these results testify to the relevance of syllabic units at the interface of phonological and phonetic encoding; however, they do not represent indisputable evidence for the notion of separately stored syllabic units. In contrast, syllable frequency effects represent strong evidence for the existence of the syllabary because only stored units are thought to exhibit frequency effects.

Both psycholinguistic and neurolinguistic studies have investigated the impact of syllable frequency on the speed and accuracy with which the stored motor programs are retrieved and overtly articulated. In analogy to the *word-frequency effect* (Jescheniak & Levelt, 1994; Oldfield & Winfield, 1965), effects of *syllable* frequency are thought to support the notion that syllables are retrieved as whole entities during the process of speech planning. In psycholinguistic studies, speakers are expected to produce high-frequency syllables faster than low-frequency syllables. The manipulated syllables are either presented as monosyllables or are embedded into multisyllabic contexts. In neurolinguistic studies, neurological patients with apraxia of speech (AOS), a neurological impairment that seems to be tied to the motor programming of syllables, are expected to produce high-frequency syllables more accurately than low-frequency syllables.

EFFECTS OF SYLLABLE FREQUENCY IN PSYCHOLINGUISTIC STUDIES

Levelt and Wheeldon (1994) were the first who attempted to identify stored syllabic units by means of syllable frequency effects in speech production. They investigated naming latencies for Dutch words consisting of high- versus low-frequency syllables. Levelt and Wheeldon's core finding was that, when word frequency was controlled for, words with high-frequency syllables were named faster than words with low-frequency syllables. If syllables are computed on-line rather than retrieved from a repository, their frequency of use should be irrelevant. Therefore, the obtained syllable frequency effects seemed to support the notion of the mental syllabary, where syllables are stored separately from words. However, in some of Levelt and Wheeldon's experiments, syllable and segment frequencies were correlated. In follow-up experiments by Levelt and Meyer (reported in Hendriks & McQueen 1996), in which a large number of possible confounding factors were controlled for, neither syllable nor segment frequency effects were obtained. Although the Levelt and Wheeldon study had some drawbacks, it formulated a clear proposal of the mental syllabary, and it highlighted the importance of controlling for potential confounds in the material set.

Another study testing the production of high- and low-frequency syllables in Dutch was carried out by Cholin, Levelt, and Schiller (2006). A symbol-position-association learning task was used to contrast the production of high- and low-frequency syllables in mono- and disyllabic pseudowords. The basic syllable material was carefully controlled for any potential confounds such as phoneme and biphone frequency, CV structure, and the transitional probabilities between the single phonemes of the syllables. The participants' task was to respond as fast as possible with a previously learned target word when a production cue was presented on the screen. The results revealed a significant syllable frequency effect with monosyllabic pseudowords. This effect was replicated investigating disyllabic pseudowords bearing the frequency manipulation on the first syllable. Because potential confounds were controlled for, these findings provide compelling evidence for the notion of a mental syllabary.

Further evidence for syllable frequency effects also comes from other languages including Spanish, French, and English. Carreiras and Perea (2004) reported syllable frequency effects in Spanish speech production tasks (see also Perea & Carreiras, 1996). In French, Brand, Rey, Peereman, and Spieler (2002) found significant syllable frequency effects in a larger-scale study. Laganaro (2003) investigated effects of syllable frequency in French and found that syllable frequency affected naming latencies in a picture-naming experiment (see also Alario, Ferrand, Laganaro, New, Frauenfelder, & Segui, 2004) and in nonword reading.

Investigations of syllable frequency in English have yielded inconsistent results. Monsell, van der Lugt, and Jessiman (2002) failed to find any differences in the rapid production of prepared utterances consisting of nonword sequences composed of frequent syllables and those composed of syllables that do not occur in English. They only found a small difference in the latency for naming visually presented syllables of these two kinds, which were matched for orthographic difficulty. The authors concluded that either there is no syllabary, or the advantage it confers to production is very small. Croot and Rastle (2004) investigated effects of syllable frequency in three experiments in English. They compared naming latencies, durational length, and spectral measurements of coarticulation for high-frequency syllables and novel syllables. Under the assumption that high-frequency syllables are stored as whole programs, Croot and Rastle predicted that those syllables should not only show shorter naming latencies but also shorter durational length due to increased coarticulation in stored syllables compared to low-frequency (assembled) syllables. The results revealed a small difference in naming latencies in the predicted direction, but it did not reach statistical significance. However, the analysis of the spectral correlates of coarticulation showed stronger coarticulatory effects for high-frequency syllables than for novel syllables.

A significant influence of syllable frequency on naming times in English was observed using the symbol-position-association learning task and a material set that was constructed following the same procedures as described in Cholin et al. (2006). Cholin, Dell, and Levelt (2008) obtained shorter naming latencies for high-frequency syllables in monosyllabic pseudowords and in disyllabic pseudowords. The difference between these findings and the findings by Croot and Rastle (2004) as well as by Monsell et al. (2002) might reflect differences in statistical power. Cholin et al. collected measurements of eight repetitions[3] per syllable, whereas the other investigators measured only one production per syllable. Another difference between the Monsell et al. study and the other two studies might have been that the high-frequency syllables were not sufficiently high frequency to evoke syllable frequency effects. In general, it might be more difficult to detect syllable frequency effects in English, a language that has relatively fuzzy syllable boundaries compared to other languages. The greater statistical power of Cholin et al.'s study might have brought these very small syllable frequency effects to light.

Studies that were specifically devoted to the question of *where* syllable frequency effects arise in the process of speech planning are discussed in Cholin & Levelt (2008) and Laganaro and Alario (2006). Cholin & Levelt (2008) used a reading version of the implicit priming paradigm to test preparation effects for high- and low-frequency syllables in Dutch. High- and low-frequency syllables were presented in homogeneous and heterogeneous sets. The first syllables of disyllabic target words were either high or low frequency. The syllables were identical in homogeneous sets and not identical in heterogeneous sets. The manipulation revealed a significant interaction between the effects of preparation and frequency. The interaction was interpreted as follows: The low-frequency syllables in homogeneous sets had a larger benefit due to preparation than high-frequency syllables, whereas high-frequency syllables were produced faster than low-frequency syllables in heterogeneous sets where no preparation was possible. This finding crucially supports the assumption that syllable frequency sensitive units are accessed after phonological encoding has been completed, thereby providing evidence for a syllable store located between the levels of phonological and phonetic encoding.

Along the same line, Laganaro and Alario (2006) manipulated syllable frequency in French to investigate where syllable frequency effects arise in speech production. They contrasted syllable frequency in word-, pseudoword-, and picture-naming studies using both immediate and delayed naming variants. They report syllable frequency effects for pseudoword and picture naming in the immediate variant, as well as for word and pseudoword naming in the delayed variant when the delay was filled with an articulatory suppression task. The authors interpret this as evidence that syllable frequency effects arise at the level of phonetic encoding. Thus, these latter two studies not only add further evidence to the claim that syllables are retrieved as whole units, they also converge on the location where the units are stored, namely at a level following phonological encoding.

In summary, there are a good number of studies using different tasks with existing words and pseudowords in different languages which support the hypothesis that syllables are independently stored units. However, the finding that high-frequency syllables are produced faster and more accurately than low-frequency syllables is neutral with respect to the existence of a potential online assembly route. The different speech onset latencies for high- and low-frequency syllables could be attributed to a (faster) retrieval for high-frequency syllables from memory and a slow(er)-operating online assembly for low-frequency syllables, but the current results could also be interpreted as showing that both high- *and* low-frequency syllables (at least the ones used in the reviewed studies) are stored. In this case, faster

---

[3] Note, however, that there was no immediate repetition of the same syllable. Participants always produced a random digit between two consecutive syllables.

latencies are an indication of faster activation for high-frequency syllables than for low-frequency syllables. The experimental comparison of novel syllables and (existing) high-frequency syllables might provide the strongest test case for a hypothesised assembly route because new syllables cannot have a match in the syllabary and must be constructed, whereas high-frequency syllables are the best candidates for storage.[4] However, the studies by Croot and Rastle (2004) and Monsell et al. (2002) did not find significant effects for this contrast. As already pointed out, the lack of statistical power might have been disadvantageous, particularly in the context of novel syllables that might have introduced too much variance into the material set. Yet another possibility could be that the system, confronted with experimental novel syllables, opted to switch entirely to an online assembly route, which would have diminished any potential difference between high-frequency syllables and novel syllables.[5] This explanation would have two implications: (a) the system can "decide" what route to employ in a given context and (b) low-frequency syllables (at least the ones that were used in the reviewed studies) are also likely to be stored within the syllabary because syllable frequency effects were obtained for these comparisons. Clearly, further research is needed in order to investigate these implications. It is fortunate that syllable frequency effects were concordantly observed in a number of studies in different languages employing different tasks, such as picture naming, word naming, reading, and learning paradigms that investigated syllables in words and pseudowords. The measurement of other syllabic parameters such as coarticulation and duration patterns can complement insights from widely used reaction time studies by providing a window into different mechanisms used to generate phonetic syllables.

EFFECTS OF SYLLABLE FREQUENCY IN NEUROLINGUISTIC STUDIES

What would be a potential result of damage to the mental syllabary? The evidence for stored (high-frequency) syllables underpins the relevance of pre-compiled whole gestural scores for the speech of healthy, neurologically intact speakers whose speech greatly benefits from the retrieval of ready-made units both in speed and accuracy. Apraxia of speech (AOS), a neurological impairment that follows from certain types of brain injury (stroke, head trauma, tumour, or other neurological diseases), might exhibit deficits that have the potential to shed light on different routes used to generate syllabic motor programs.

Patients with AOS have been described as being unable to produce the correct sounds of words in the proper sequence with the appropriate timing while not exhibiting any significant impairment of speech comprehension, reading, or writing, or any significant paralysis or weakness of the speech musculature (Dronkers, 1996; Lebrun, 1990). Many authors have argued that speech apraxia is caused by the distortion of the transfer between phonological and phonetic encoding processes

---

[4] Notice, however, that the classification of novel syllables relies almost exclusively on databases that respect word boundaries. It therefore seems conceivable that the frequency of syllables is underestimated because (re)syllabification across word boundaries is not taken into account. For example, the occurrence of the syllable "dit" in the spoken context of "de.fen.dit" is not captured within databases.

[5] The fact that there were twice as many novel syllables as existing syllables in Experiment 2 of the Croot and Rastle (2004) study might have added to this effect.

(Code, 1998; Nickels & Howard, 2000; Varley & Whiteside, 2001a; Ziegler, 2002, see also Gandour, Petty, & Dardarananda, 1989; Kent & Rosenbek, 1983; and for an overview see Whiteside & Varley, 1998, 2001a). Furthermore, it has been argued that deficits described as characteristic for AOS are caused by an impaired access to stored syllables in a mental syllabary (Varley & Whiteside, 2001a, 2001b; Varley, Whiteside, & Luff, 1999).

Thus, if we assume that the pathomechanism of AOS is located at the interface of phonological and phonetic encoding where access to the mental syllabary is assumed to take place, the following predictions can be made: (1) If access to the mental syllabary is in fact impaired in these patients, one would expect that syllable frequency effects vanish or are at least reduced: High-frequency syllables should no longer have an advantage over low-frequency syllables if both types of syllables need to be assembled online. (2) If access to the syllabary is still preserved, one would expect the high-frequency syllables to be less impaired than the low-frequency syllables and the syllable frequency effect might be even more pronounced. A related prediction could be made under the assumption that speech apraxia results from an inability to *assemble* syllable programs. If that is in fact the case, then the production of *stored* high-frequency syllables should be easier.

Varley et al. (1999) and Varley and Whiteside (2001a, 2001b) specifically proposed that AOS can be explained in part by an impaired access to the mental syllabary that in turn forces patients with AOS to generate syllables by means of an alternative "segment-by-segment" route. Varley et al. (1999) used a word-repetition task to compare the production latencies and durations of monosyllabic high- and low-frequency words embedded in noun phrases to compare the production latencies of patients with AOS, aphasic patients, and neurologically intact speakers. They predicted, following the "dual route" hypothesis, that patients with AOS should not show a frequency effect because the frequency sensitive route via the mental syllabary is impaired. In other words, the assembly of high-frequency words should be as effortful as the assembly of low-frequency ones. The results were in favour of this hypothesis: Whereas high-frequency words were spoken more quickly (shorter response latencies) and with shorter durations in the group of aphasic patients and the control group, there was no such effect in the AOS group. However, contrary to the Levelt et al. notion of a mental syllabary, Varley et al. (1999) assume that speakers have access to a store that contains motor programs for *word* forms rather than for syllables. Accordingly, they tested existing monosyllabic words and controlled for word frequency instead of syllable frequency. The correlation and potential interaction of word and frequency is not traceable. Thus, this result cannot be taken as evidence for or against the prediction that patients with AOS have to rely on an online assembly that generates *syllables*.

A study that tested Varley and Whiteside's dual-route hypothesis more appropriately—namely the prediction that patients with AOS have lost access to the mental syllabary—was conducted by Aichert and Ziegler (2004) using item lists manipulating *syllable* frequency and syllable structure in German in patients with mild and severe AOS. In order to specifically test the claim that patients with AOS have to rely on an online assembly route, two *syllabic* parameters within disyllabic words were separately manipulated and tested in a word repetition task. The first manipulation concerned the (high or low) frequency of the first syllable in an overall low-frequency disyllabic word. Syllables in this list were controlled for CV structure. The second manipulation was based on the finding that patients with AOS tend to simplify consonant clusters into one segment (McNeil, Liss, Tseng, & Kent, 1990; Odell, McNeil, Rosenbek, & Hunter, 1990). If the pathomechanism underlying AOS is devoted to syllables rather than words, consonant clusters within a syllable—that is, in onset (CCVC) or coda position (CVCC) in monosyllabic words—should be more vulnerable than clusters that occur across syllable boundaries (CVC.CV) in disyllabic words. Both of the syllabic manipulations revealed interesting outcomes: The manipulation of syllable frequency had a significant influence on error rates in both patient groups: patients with mild AOS showed virtually no errors on the high-frequency syllables but did produce errors on the low-frequency syllables, while the patients with severe AOS produced errors even on the high-frequency syllables and showed a further increase of error rates on the low-frequency syllables. The finding of a frequency effect on error rates speaks against the assumption that patients with AOS suffer from an impaired access to the mental syllabary, as suggested by Varley and colleagues. The additional manipulation of syllable structure showed that both patient groups reduced consonant clusters within a syllable more often than within a word (i.e., the total of onset and coda simplification was significantly higher than the cluster reductions across a syllable boundary), which strengthens the assumption that the pathomechanism underlying AOS is in fact sensitive to syllables (rather than words).

How can these findings be explained against the background of the mental syllabary theory and the hypothesis that patients with AOS have lost access to the mental syllabary? As Aichert and Ziegler (2004) conclude, the current results are difficult to explain with the hypothesis that AOS speakers have lost access to stored syllables. If the deficit causing AOS forces these patients to rely (entirely) on a (segment-by-segment) online assembly route, no frequency effects should have been obtained because high-frequency syllables should have no advantage in their assembly compared to low-frequency syllables. The finding that patients with mild AOS show virtually no errors on syllables within the highest frequency range, but produced significantly more errors on syllables with lower frequency, suggests that these patients do have access to the syllabary, at least to the most high-frequency syllables. As stated above, it seems likely that early acquired, highly overused syllables form the core of the syllabary and might be less vulnerable than less frequent syllables (and possibly smaller units), which are perhaps less anchored within the syllabary. Patients with severe AOS might have lost access to the syllabary or, as suggested by Aichert and Ziegler (2004), their access might be preserved but the syllabic entries themselves are damaged. In this case, whether defective syllables are generally disregarded and replaced by online-assembled syllables or retrieved and articulated without further modifications, remains an open question.

Taken together, Varley and Whiteside's (2001a) claim that patients with AOS are forced to compensate for lost access to the syllabary by generating motor programs for syllables via an online segment-by-segment route seems unsustainable, at least in this strict interpretation. The underlying deficit of AOS might in part be explained by a loss of stored motor programs, but the assumption of a complete reliance on an online segment-by-segment route in AOS (and, thus, evidence in favour of a dual-route system) is not supported by a better-suited investigation of syllabic parameters (such as syllable frequency and syllable structure) in the study by Aichert and Ziegler (2004). These results do not rule out the possibility that speakers do, in fact, have an alternative route at their disposal, but it clearly indicates that this is not the only route operating in AOS.

SUMMARY AND OUTLOOK

This article reviewed investigations with both neurologically intact speakers and neurological patients who suffer from AOS, a deficit that has been located at the level where unimpaired speakers access stored motor programs for syllables. An issue that has accompanied the investigations of the mental syllabary and the search for indisputable evidence for independently stored units is the question of whether or not there is an alternative mechanism that operates alongside the retrieval route. Undoubtedly, speakers must have a mechanism that allows them to construct motor programs for syllables they have never encountered before. The question at hand is whether there is, in fact, an additional assembly route that constructs phonetic syllables segment by segment, (see Levelt, 1989; Levelt et al. 1999; Varley & Whiteside, 2001a) or whether there is *no* additional route but rather an additional *mechanism* that operates within the syllabary. This mechanism could produce a syllable that is not stored as such in the syllabary by addressing smaller units such as demisyllables, onsets, and rhymes, which might also be part of the stored inventory. These smaller units would then be integrated into one joint syllable during a subsequent encoding step. If and how these subsyllabic parts are integrated into a syllable context and how the frequencies of the subsyllabic parts interact with the syllable frequencies remains subject to further research. Unequivocally, the core of the mental syllabary consists of early-acquired, high-frequency syllables that are embedded in a network with syllabic neighbours; the number of these high-frequency syllables might be correctly estimated at 500 syllables (Schiller et al., 1996). Although it cannot be excluded that *all* syllables, once produced, will find their copy in the syllabary, it seems unlikely that all of the remaining 11,000 to 12,000 syllables (the total number of syllables in languages such as English, Dutch, and German) are stored. However, every one of these syllables could potentially be stored, at least temporarily. Ultimately, the frequency of any given unit might be the decisive criterion for a potential storage within the mental syllabary. We can only speculate how new syllables are acquired (or re-acquired, see Aichert & Ziegler, 2008 this issue) and how they might find their gestural mapping over repeated use.[6] While factors such as frequency, *age of acquisition* and *neighbourhood density* (see Vitevitch, 2002, Vitevitch, Armbruster, & Chu, 2004; Vitevitch & Sommers, 2003) can possibly tell us more about the internal organisation of the syllabary, measurements of coarticulatory and durational patterns might offer further insights into the inherent structure of syllables with different frequencies. So far, neither the psycholinguistic nor the neurolinguistic studies provide undisputable evidence in support of an online segment-by-segment assembly route. The existence of a mental syllabary that

---

[6] It is an empirical question how multiple repetitions of the same syllable motor program might diminish a potential frequency effect and might potentially result in a stored entry in the syllabary. The pilot study in Cholin (2004) in which participants produced high- and low-frequency syllables multiple times in the practice phase revealed no syllable frequency effect in the actual experiment. Thus, practice seems to have a rapid impact on the frequency status of syllables. Notice, however, that eight repetitions of the same syllable still show a detectable difference in the voice onset latencies for high- and low-frequency syllables (Cholin et al, 2006; Cholin et al., 2008).

contains (at least) the high-frequency syllables of a speaker's language seems to have been proven by the available psycholinguistic and neurolinguistic data. The faster production of high-frequency syllables in reaction time experiments on the one hand, and the more accurate production of these syllables in patients with AOS on the other hand, converge on this point. In this sense, the joint analysis of these two lines of research offers not only two approaches to test specific predictions but also potential insights into the impaired and unimpaired processes of language production, in particular into the levels of phonological and phonetic encoding. In order to further investigate details of phonetic encoding, other methods, such as brain-imaging techniques (e.g., Dogil et al., 2002) could potentially add to our understanding of stored and computed phonetic units. The integration of these different approaches and domains seems most promising to develop a common framework for fluent speech production as well as for the non-fluent, impaired speech production.

REFERENCES

Aichert, I., & Ziegler, W. (2004). Syllable frequency and syllable structure in apraxia of speech. *Brain and Language, 88*, 148–159.

Aichert, I., & Ziegler, W. (2008). Learning a syllable from its parts: Cross-syllabic generalisation effects in patients with apraxia of speech. *Aphasiology, 22*, 1216–1229.

Alario, F-X., Ferrand, L., Laganaro, M., New, B., Frauenfelder, U. H., & Segui, J. (2004). Predictors of picture naming speed. *Behavior Research Methods Instruments & Computers, 36*, 140–155.

Baumann, M. (1995). *The production of syllables in connected speech.* PhD dissertation, Nijmegen University, the Netherlands.

Booij, G. (1995). *The phonology of Dutch.* Oxford, UK: Clarendon Press.

Brand, M., Rey, A., & Peereman, R. (2003). Where is the syllable priming effect in visual word recognition? *Journal of Memory and Language, 48*, 435–443.

Brand, M., Rey, A., Peereman, R., & Spieler, D. (2002). Naming bisyllabic words: A large scale study. *Abstracts of the Psychonomic Society, 7*, 94.

Browman, C. P., & Goldstein, L. (1988). Some notes on syllable structure in articulatory phonology. *Phonetica, 45*, 140–155.

Browman, C. P., & Goldstein, L. (1992a). Articulatory phonology: An overview. *Phonetica, 49*, 155–180.

Buxbaum, L. J., & Coslett, H. B. (2001). Spatio-motor aspects of action. In B. Rapp (Ed.), *The handbook of cognitive neuropsychology* (pp. 543–563). Philadelphia: Psychology Press.

Buxbaum, L. J., Kyle, K. M., & Menon, R. (2005). On beyond mirror neurons: Internal representations subserving imitation and recognition of skilled object-related actions in humans. *Brain Research, 25*, 226–239.

Byrd, D. (1995). C-centers revisited. *Phonetica, 52*, 285–306.

Byrd, D. (1996). Influences on articulatory timing in consonant sequences. *Journal of Phonetics, 24*, 209–244.

Carreiras, M., & Perea, M. (2004). Naming pseudowords in Spanish: Effects of syllable frequency in production. *Brain and Language, 90*, 393–400.

Chen, J-Y., Lin, W-C., & Ferrand, L. (2003). Masked priming of the syllable in Mandarin Chinese speech production. *Chinese Journal of Psychology, 45*, 107–120.

Cholin, J. (2004). *The syllable in speech production. Effects of syllable preparation and syllable frequency.* PhD dissertation, Radboud University Nijmegen, the Netherlands (MPI series 26).

Cholin, J., Dell, G. S., & Levelt, W. J. M. (2008). *The coordination of planning and articulation procedures in incremental speech production.* Manuscript in preparation.

Cholin, J., Levelt, W. J. M., & Schiller, N. O. (2006). Effects of syllable frequency in speech production. *Cognition, 50*, 205–235.

Cholin, J., & Levelt, W. J. M. (2008). *Effects of syllable preparation and syllable frequency in speech production: Further evidence for the retrieval of stored syllables at a post-lexical level.* Manuscript submitted for publication.

Cholin, J., Schiller, N. O., & Levelt, W. J. M. (2004). The preparation of syllables in speech production. *Journal of Memory and Language, 50*, 47–61.

Code, C. (1998). Major review: Models, theories and heuristics in apraxia of speech. *Clinical Linguistics and Phonetics, 12*, 47–65.

Costa, A., & Sebastián-Gallés, N. (1998). Abstract phonological structure in language production: Evidence from Spanish. *Journal of Experimental Psychology: Learning, Memory and Cognition, 24*, 886–903.

Croot, K., & Rastle, K. (2004). *Is there a syllabary containing stored articulatory plans for speech production in English?*. Proceedings of the 10th Australian International Conference on Speech Science and Technology, Macquarie University, Sydney, 8–10 December.

Dell, G. S. (1986). A spreading-activation theory of retrieval in sentence production. *Psychological Review, 93*, 283–321.

Dell, G. S. (1988). The retrieval of phonological forms in production: Tests of predictions from a connectionist model. *Journal of Memory and Language, 27*, 124–142.

Dogil, G., Riecker, A., Ackermann, H., Wildgruber, Mayer, J., & Haider, H. et al. (2002). The speaking brain: A tutorial introduction to fMRI experiments in the production of speech, prosody and syntax. *Journal of Neurolinguistics, 15*, 59–90.

Dronkers, N. F. (1996). A new brain region for coordinating speech articulation. *Nature, 384*, 159–161.

Evinck, S. (1997). *Production de la parole en français: Investigation des unités impliquées dans l'encodage phonologique des mots* [Speech production in French: Investigation of the units implied during the phonological encoding of words]. Unpublished PhD dissertation, Bruxelles University, Belgium.

Farnetani, E. (1990). V-C-V lingual coarticulation and its spatiotemporal domain. In W. J. Hardcastle & A. Marchal (Eds.), *Speech production and speech modelling* (pp. 93–130). Dordrecht: Kluwer.

Ferrand, L., Segui, J., & Grainger, J. (1996). Masked priming of word and picture naming: The role of syllable units. *Journal of Memory and Language, 35*, 708–723.

Ferrand, L., Segui, J., & Humphreys, G. W. (1997). The syllable's role in word naming. *Memory & Cognition, 25*, 458–470.

Gandour, J., Petty, S. H., & Dardarananda, R. (1989). Dysprosody in Broca's aphasia: A case study. *Brain and Language, 37*, 232–257.

Goldstein, L., & Fowler, C. A. (2003). Articulatory phonology: A phonology for public language use. In N. O. Schiller & A. S. Meyer (Eds.), *Phonetics and phonology in language comprehension and production: Differences and similarities* (pp. 159–207). Berlin: Mouton de Gruyter.

Hendriks, H., & McQueen, J. (Eds.). (1996). *Annual Report 1995*. Max Planck Institute for Psycholinguistics, Nijmegen, the Netherlands.

Indefrey, P., & Levelt, W. J. M. (2000). The neural correlates of languages production. In M. Gazzaniga (Ed.), *The new cognitive neurosciences* (pp. 845–865). Cambridge, MA: MIT Press.

Jescheniak, J. D., & Levelt, W. J. M. (1994). Word frequency effects in speech production: Retrieval of syntactic information and of phonological form. *Journal of Experimental Psychology: Learning, Memory, and Cognition, 20*, 824–843.

Kent, R., & Rosenbek, J. (1983). Acoustic patterns of apraxia of speech. *Journal of Speech and Hearing Research, 26*, 231–249.

Kerzel, D., & Bekkering, H. (2000). Motor activation from visible speech: Evidence from stimulus–response compatibility. *Journal of Experimental Psychology: Human Perception and Performance, 26*, 634–647.

Laganaro, M. (2003). *Are syllables represented and retrieved during phonological encoding? An integration of psycholinguistic and neurolinguistic studies.* Poster presented at Euresco conference on The Science of Aphasia: Functional Neuroimaging Studies of Language and its Impairments. Italy: Acquafredda di Maratea.

Laganaro, M., & Alario, F-X. (2006). On the locus of the syllable frequency effect in language production. *Journal of Memory and Language, 55*, 178–196.

Lebrun, Y. (1990). Apraxia of speech: A critical review. *Journal of Neurolinguistics, 5*, 379–406.

Levelt, W. J. M. (1989). *Speaking. From intention to articulation.* Cambridge, MA: MIT Press.

Levelt, W. J. M. (1992). Accessing words in speech production: Stages, processes and representations. *Cognition, 42*, 1–22.

Levelt, W. J. M. (2001). Spoken word production: A theory of lexical access. *Proceedings of the National Academy of Sciences, 98*, 13464–13471.

Levelt, W. J. M., Roelofs, A., & Meyer, A. S. (1999). A theory of lexical access in speech production. *Behavioral and Brain Sciences, 22*, 1–75.

Levelt, W. J. M., & Wheeldon, L. (1994). Do speakers have access to a mental syllabary? *Cognition, 50*, 239–269.

McNeil, M. R., Liss, J. M., Tseng, C. H., & Kent, R. D. (1990). Effects of speech rate on the absolute and relative timing of apraxic and conduction aphasic sentence production. *Brain and Language, 38*, 135–158.

Meyer, A. S. (1990). The time course of phonological encoding in language production: The encoding of successive syllables of a word. *Journal of Memory and Language, 29*, 524–545.

Meyer, A. S. (1991). The time course of phonological encoding in language production: Phonological encoding inside a syllable. *Journal of Memory and Language, 30*, 69–89.

Miller, N. (2001). Dual or duel route? *Aphasiology, 15*, 62–68.

Monsell, S., van der Lugt, A., & Jessiman, T. (2002, April). *In pursuit of the syllabary: This Snark is a Boojum!*. Paper presented at the Experimental Psychology Society Meeting, Leuven, Belgium.

Nickels, L., & Howard, D. (2000). *When the words won't come: Relating impairments and models of spoken word production*. In L. Wheeldon (Ed.), *Aspects of language production* (pp. 115–142). Hove, UK: Psychology Press.

Odell, K., McNeil, M. R., Rosenbek, J. C., & Hunter, L. (1990). Perceptual characteristics of consonant production by apraxic speakers. *Journal of Speech and Hearing Disorders, 55*, 345–359.

Oldfield, R. C., & Wingfield, A. (1965). Response latencies in naming objects. *Quarterly Journal of Experimental Psychology, 17*, 273–281.

Perea, M., & Carreiras, M. (1996). Efectos de frecuencia silábica en la tarea de pronunciación mixta [Effects of syllable frequency in the mixed pronunciation task]. *Psicológica, 17*, 425–440.

Recasens, D. (1984). V-to-C coarticulation in Catalan VCV sequences: An articulatory and acoustic study. *Journal of Phonetics, 12*, 61–73.

Recasens, D. (1987). An acoustic analysis of V-to-C and V-to-V coarticulatory effects in Catalan and Spanish VCV sequences. *Journal of Phonetics, 15*, 299–312.

Roelofs, A. (1992). A spreading-activation theory of lemma retrieval in speaking. *Cognition, 42*, 107–142.

Roelofs, A. (1997a). Syllabification in speech production: Evaluation of WEAVER. *Language and Cognitive Processes, 12*, 657–693.

Roelofs, A. (1997b). The WEAVER model of word form encoding in speech production. *Cognition, 64*, 249–284.

Roelofs, A. (1999). Phonological segments and features as planning units in speech production. *Language and Cognitive Processes, 14*, 173–200.

Roelofs, A. (2002a). Syllable structure effects turn out to be word length effects; Comment on Santiago et al. (2000). *Language and Cognitive Processes, 17*, 1–13.

Roelofs, A. (2002b). Storage and computation in spoken word production. In S. Nooteboom, F. Weerman, & F. Wijnen (Eds.), *Storage and computation in the language faculty* (pp. 183–216). Dordrecht: Kluwer.

Saltzman, E. (1986). Task dynamic coordination of the speech articulators: A preliminary model. In H. Heuer & C. Fromm (Eds.), *Generation and modulation of action patterns*. [Experimental Brain Research series 15, pp. 129–144]. New York: Springer-Verlag.

Saltzman, E., & Kelso, J. A. S. (1987). Skilled actions: A task-dynamic approach. *Psychological Review, 94*, 84–106.

Schiller, N. O. (1998). The effect of visually masked primes on the naming latencies of words and pictures. *Journal of Memory and Language, 39*, 484–507.

Schiller, N. O. (1999). Masked syllable priming of English nouns. *Brain and Language, 68*, 300–305.

Schiller, N. O. (2000). Single word production in English: The role of subsyllabic units during speech production. *Journal of Experimental Psychology: Learning, Memory and Cognition, 26*, 512–528.

Schiller, N. O. (2004). The onset effect in word naming. *Journal of Memory and Language, 50*, 477–490.

Schiller, N. O., & Costa, A. (2006). Activation of segments, not syllables, during phonological encoding in speech production. *The Mental Lexicon, 1*, 231–250.

Schiller, N. O., Costa, A., & Colomé, A. (2002). Phonological encoding of single words: In search of the lost syllable. In C. Gussenhoven & N. Warner (Eds.), *Papers in laboratory phonology 7* (pp. 35–59). Berlin: Mouton de Gruyter.

Schiller, N. O., Meyer, A. S., Baayen, R. H., & Levelt, W. J. M. (1996). A comparison of lexeme and speech syllables in Dutch. *Journal of Quantitative Linguistics, 3*, 8–28.

Schiller, N. O., Meyer, A. S., & Levelt, W. J. M. (1997). The syllabic structure of spoken words: Evidence from the syllabification of intervocalic consonants. *Language and Speech, 40*, 103–140.

Sevald, C. A., Dell, G., & Cole, J. S. (1995). Syllable structure in speech production: Are syllables chunks or schemas? *Journal of Memory and Language, 34*, 807–820.

Varley, R., & Whiteside, S. (2001a). What is the underlying impairment in acquired apraxia of speech. *Aphasiology, 15*, 39–49.

Varley, R., & Whiteside, S. (2001b). Exploring the enigma. *Aphasiology, 15*, 78–84.

Varley, R., Whiteside, S., & Luff, H. (1999). Apraxia of speech as a disruption of word-level schemata: Some durational evidence. *Journal of Medical Speech-Language Pathology, 7*, 127–132.

Vitevitch, M. S. (2002). The influence of phonological similarity neighborhoods on speech production. *Journal of Experimental Psychology: Learning, Memory, & Cognition, 28*, 735–747.

Vitevitch, M. S., Armbruster, J., & Chu, S. (2004). Sub-lexical and lexical representations in speech production: Effects of phonotactic probability and onset density. *Journal of Experimental Psychology: Learning, Memory, & Cognition, 30*, 514–529.

Vitevitch, M. S., & Sommers, M. (2003). The facilitative influence of phonological similarity and neighborhood frequency in speech production. *Memory & Cognition, 31*, 491–504.

Whiteside, S. P., & Varley, R. A. (1998). A reconceptualisation of apraxia of speech: A synthesis of evidence. *Cortex, 34*, 221–231.

Ziegler, W. (2002). Psycholinguistic and motor theories of apraxia of speech. *Seminars in Speech and Language, 23*, 231–243.

Ziegler, W., Thelen, A-K., Staiger, A., & Liepold, M. (2008). The domain of phonetic encoding in apraxia of speech: Which sub-lexical units count? *Aphasiology, 22*, 1230–1247.

APHASIOLOGY, 2008, 22 (11), 1142–1156

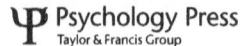

Sublexical units in aphasic jargon and in the standard language: Comparative analyses of neologisms in connected speech

Prisca Stenneken

Clinical Linguistics Unit, University of Bielefeld, and Freie Universität Berlin, Germany

Markus J. Hofmann and Arthur M. Jacobs

Freie Universität Berlin, Germany

Background: It is a well-documented finding that phonemic speech errors in aphasia reflect certain characteristics of their intended targets. However, only few studies have investigated spontaneous speech productions of jargon-aphasic patients, in which lexical targets may be completely unrecognisable (abstruse phonemic neologisms). There is some evidence that these neologisms correspond to the standard language concerning phonemic content and structure.

Aims: The present study further explores similarities of aphasic neologisms and the standard language, to contribute to the discussion about the origin of non-target-related errors in jargon aphasia. It investigates whether similarities at the phoneme level can be confirmed even in connected, severely jargonised speech that does not allow identification of lexical targets. Moreover, it raises the question whether other sublexical units like syllables contribute to the formation of phonemic neologisms.

Methods & Procedures: Neologisms in spontaneous speech of a German-speaking jargon-aphasic patient were compared to the standard language concerning phoneme and syllable inventory, structural aspects, and distributional frequencies of sublexical measures. Data of the standard language were derived from meta-analyses of a German phonological word form database.

Outcomes & Results: A strong relatedness to the standard language was demonstrated for the aphasic neologisms in connected speech. Similarities regarded phoneme inventory, phonotactics, and phoneme frequency distributions. The patient data point to a preferred use of high-frequency phonemes and syllables in neologisms. In addition, a similar distribution of syllable frequencies and structures was observed in the neologisms and in standard German. Results indicate that syllable frequency serves as a predictor for the neologisms' distributional frequencies.

Conclusions: The present study indicated that phonemic neologisms with no or weak evidence for a lexical origin still conformed to the phonological characteristics of the standard language, suggesting undisturbed segmental phonological processing. With respect to processing levels in speech production, results specifically pointed to a prominent role of syllabic units. The present findings are compatible with the assumption that syllabic representations, like structural information of syllables, are constrained in neologism formation.

Keywords: Jargon aphasia; Neologism; Syllable frequency; Phoneme frequency; Syllable structure.

Address correspondence to: Prisca Stenneken, Clinical Linguistics Unit, University of Bielefeld, Postfach 10 01 31, 33501 Bielefeld, Germany. E-mail: prisca.stenneken@uni-bielefeld.de

http://www.psypress.com/aphasiology   DOI: 10.1080/02687030701820501

Speech production in jargon aphasia is typically characterised by frequent occurrence of neologistic utterances, and thus often involves a severe impairment in conveying lexical meaning. The neologistic, nonword utterances deviate from the standard language in their phonemic or semantic properties, making it difficult or impossible to identify lexical content (phonemic or semantic neologisms). With regard to phonemic neologisms, which are the focus of the present study, a distinction between two subtypes of jargon has been suggested. In neologistic jargon the nonword utterances are embedded into identifiable words or phrases, whereas phonemic jargon consists almost entirely of nonword utterances (Butterworth, 1985). Common to different forms of jargon aphasia is the observation that patients show fluent speech production, often accompanied by an auditory comprehension deficit and a failure to monitor their speech output (overview in Marshall, 2006).

Previous studies of phonemic errors in jargon have focused on the question of how far the nonword errors are related to their intended lexical targets.[1] This has been a key issue in the debate concerning the origin of aphasic jargon. Findings of a high degree of target-relatedness in nonword errors (e.g., Dell, Schwartz, Martin, Saffran, & Gagnon, 1997; Hillis, Boatman, Hart, & Gordon, 1999) have been taken to demonstrate a lexical involvement in the neologistic productions. Thus, if similarities to the target form can be identified, the nonword error is assumed to arise from at least partial access to the target's lexical–phonological information (target-related error). Jargon-aphasic utterances that do not allow identification of lexical targets (so-called abstruse neologisms; Lecours, 1982) have been empirically investigated less often. This may be attributed to the relatively rarer occurrence of cases with abstruse neologism production and to the methodological challenges of having no direct comparative data set when no targets can be identified. Still, non-target-related errors, in which the degree of lexical involvement is less obvious, present a theoretically most interesting case for investigating the processing levels that are relevant for neologism generation. In spite of the unidentifiable lexical content, jargon-aphasic speech may reflect certain characteristics of the standard language, pointing to unimpaired processing.

In general, similarities to the standard language have been reported for supralexical as well as sublexical structures in jargon. At the supralexical level, these concern normal prosodic contours and syntactic compositions (Dogil, Hildebrandt, & Schürmeier, 1990; Duchan, Stengel, & Oliva, 1980). At the sublexical level, jargon-aphasic errors have been repeatedly described to show a normal phoneme inventory and correspond to the phonotactic constraints of the standard language (overview in Marshall, 2006). However, the phonemic similarity between aphasic neologisms and the standard language is not undisputed (cf. Butterworth, 1979; Perecman & Brown, 1981; Peuser & Temp, 1981). Peuser and Temp (1981) have pointed to deviations in phoneme frequency distributions when comparing the seven most frequent phonemes of an English-speaking jargon-aphasic patient to the seven most frequent phonemes in standard English. Although these results argue

---

[1] The terminology concerning nonword errors in jargon aphasia, including neologisms and phonemic paraphasias, has not been used consistently in previous studies, especially with regard to the underlying impairment. Where no clear distinction between neologisms as non-target-related errors and phonemic paraphasias as target-related errors is made, the present study will refer to the descriptive category of *nonword errors*. Also, in the scope of the present study, we will use the term *jargon* to refer only to phonologically distorted utterances in neologistic or phonemic jargon aphasia, excluding semantic jargon.

against a one-to-one correspondence in frequency ranks, the findings do not exclude a general similarity in frequency distributions. In other cases, phonemes that are not part of the standard language might also be observed when jargon aphasia is accompanied by articulatory or speech impairments. Besides, deviations in phoneme frequency distributions can occur if the aphasic jargon contains recurring utterances or repetition phenomena (a common feature of jargon), resulting in the over-proportionate use of single phonemes which in turn would mask phonemic similarities to the standard language.

Concerning the empirical investigation of similarities between aphasic neologisms and the standard language, not many studies have directly addressed distributional frequencies of sublexical units. Two studies of English-speaking patients have suggested that the frequency of occurrence for phonemes reflected the phoneme frequency distribution in standard English (Hanlon & Edmondson, 1996; Robson, Pring, Marshall, & Chiat, 2003). With regard to syllabic processing, studies of aphasic jargon so far have focused on the sonority structures of syllables. Analyses addressed the sonority class of phonemic segments in onset and coda positions, based on the theoretical considerations of Clements (1990). Results of non-target-related neologisms implied that the frequency distributions of sonority structures in neologisms conformed to predictions derived from theoretic frameworks (Christman, 1992, based on the English-speaking patients MS, HV, EP) and to database corpora of the standard language (Stenneken, Bastiaanse, Huber, & Jacobs, 2005a, based on the German-speaking patient KP). Whereas these findings were restricted to sonority structures in syllables, to our knowledge no studies are available so far that address individual syllables and their distributional frequencies.

To account for the frequent occurrence of non-target-related errors in aphasic jargon, it has been proposed that these nonword errors arise from a failure or impairment of lexical retrieval. In the case of blocked lexical retrieval, a qualitatively different, non-lexical source of nonword generation has been proposed (Buckingham, 1990; Butterworth, 1979; Kohn, Smith, & Alexander, 1996). The resulting utterance is regarded as a substitute form for the lexical target in connected speech. Observations that the segmental structure of the nonword errors corresponded to that of real words of the standard language have been attributed to a generation mechanism that reflects the language system's inherent properties.

Under conditions of (partial) access to the target form, the nonword errors should reflect lexical content and thus also show properties of the standard language. In addition, lexical access could be followed by a severe distortion of phonemic content, involving comparable mechanisms that underlie the production of phonemic paraphasias, i.e., the addition, elision and/or substitution of one or more phonemes. It has been suggested that these distortion mechanisms could also act on an already distorted lexical retrieval and thus produce non-target-related errors (dual impairment; cf. conduction theory, Kertesz & Benson, 1970).

Based on these considerations, the present study addressed the question of how far the non-target-related utterances in jargon aphasia reflect the characteristics of the standard language system. More specifically, the following questions were addressed: Are similarities only observed in conforming to the restrictions on phonemes and phonotactics, or is this similarity also reflected in frequency distributions? Do similarities arise at the segmental level of phonological processing, as suggested by previous studies? Or can other relevant sublexical units, like syllables, be identified, which reflect the properties of the standard language? To further explore possible post-lexical generation mechanisms for neologistic utterances, the present study compared phonemic and syllabic units in aphasic neologisms to those in the standard language. Analyses were based on neologistic utterances from the spontaneous speech production of the jargon-aphasic patient KP. This patient has been reported previously (Stenneken et al., 2005a), however, besides the different scope of the two studies, the present analyses were based on a different, larger data set. The present study reviews earlier results and discusses novel findings from KP. The relevant sublexical measures of the standard language were provided by a previous analysis of sublexical units in German (Hofmann, Stenneken, Conrad, & Jacobs, 2007).

METHOD

Case description

The patient KP, a right-handed male and monolingual native German speaker, showed jargon aphasia with a frequent production of phonemic neologisms. At the age of 59 years he suffered a CVA (thrombo-embolic stroke) of the left middle cerebral artery. CT scans revealed an extensive lesion in the perfusion region of the left middle cerebral artery reaching to occipital structures. More specific case details of the patient KP have been reported previously (Stenneken et al., 2005a).

According to standardised language testing (Aachen Aphasia Test Battery; Huber, Poeck, Weniger, & Willmes, 1983), KP's condition remained stable (testing at 5.5 and 7.5 months post-onset) and was characterised as Wernicke's aphasia with jargon. Structured language testing at 7.5 months post-onset revealed the following profile: The subtest of language comprehension was only moderately impaired, whereas severe impairments were present in all other subtests, i.e., token test, repetition, written language, and naming. There was no evidence for a speech disorder or for articulatory impairments (cf. Stenneken et al., 2005a). Accompanying deficits were ideomotor apraxia, mild right-sided facial paresis, and reduced sensibility for the right body half. Neuropsychological testing revealed deficits in visual processing and impairments in memory, learning, and attentional functions.

At the time of data collection, 7 months post-onset, spontaneous speech was fluent and utterances were interspersed with unintelligible passages. KP's speech production was characterised by the frequent occurrence of phonemic neologisms, very few phonemic paraphasias, and very rarely semantic errors. Spontaneous speech production was characterised as neologistic jargon. Here phonemic neologisms, which did not allow identifying lexical content, were embedded in short passages of intelligible speech. In contrast, KP's reading aloud was characterised as phonemic jargon, as his utterances were composed entirely of neologisms, making it impossible to identify word boundaries. In both spontaneous speech and reading aloud, KP's speech production was fluent and the intonational structure seemed adequate for German. No spontaneous self-corrections of speech errors or lexical search phenomena were observed and the patient showed no awareness that passages in his speech were incomprehensible. The identifiable utterances in KP's connected speech predominantly consisted of high-frequency function words, whereas nonword errors tended to be produced in slots in which content words would be expected. Examples of KP's neologistic utterances are [vʊt], ['keːs-bak], [gə-'veː-nəlt], often embedded in passages of intelligible phrases like "it was very ...", "and then we had ...", "that was my ...". Nonword errors were variable in their phonological forms, and perseverations of segments in successive syllables occurred only very rarely and no direct repetitions of neologistic syllables were observed. Nor was there any evidence for recurring utterances or utterances with a strong phonological relation to neighbouring productions. Previous analyses of KP's picture-naming performance (Stenneken et al., 2005a) supported that there was no clear evidence for a target-relatedness in KP's nonword errors. No systematic segmental correspondences between neologistic utterances and targets were observed concerning the overall number of phonemes or syllables and shared units of response and target. Thus, the neologistic jargon of KP provided a suitable data set for analyses of non-target-related errors, in which influences of lexical target forms and of neighbouring utterances were minimised.

Procedure

Speech data of KP were collected on two consecutive days in two sessions of about 1 hour each. Neologisms were elicited in guided spontaneous speech samples in a semi-structured interview on familiar themes and in descriptions of coloured drawings of everyday situations. The conversation was tape recorded and transcribed orthographically. All utterances that deviated from standard German (nonword errors) were phonetically transcribed by one trained coder and checked for accuracy by two others. The nonword utterances, enclosed in utterances of intelligible speech, had a length of one to three syllables. Sublexical frequency measures for KP's neologistic utterances were determined for single and dual phonemic units (phonemes and biphonemes), and for syllabic units, by summing up the frequency of occurrence for each of the units in the sample of neologistic utterances. Type frequency measures were calculated by counting the amount of words containing the respective phonemic or syllabic unit. For example, the type frequency of the syllable "ba" denotes the number of utterances that contain this unit as a syllable. In order to compare the characteristics of the aphasic errors to the standard language, the German CELEX phonological word form database (Baayen, Piepenbrock, & Gulikers, 1995) was selected as a reference base. Sublexical frequency measures of the standard language were computed for phonemes, biphonemes, and syllables (according to Hofmann et al., 2007). In addition, token frequencies were computed by summing up the lexical frequencies of the words that contain the respective sublexical unit. For example, token frequencies for the syllable "ba" were determined by adding up the word frequencies for all words possessing the syllable "ba". Lexical frequency measures were taken from the CELEX's Mannheim frequency counts in words per 6 million. All following analyses of the standard language are based on the token frequencies of the sublexical measures. More detailed information about corpus analyses and applied algorithms can be examined elsewhere (Hofmann et al., 2007). Preliminary analyses of a smaller subset of data from KP's spontaneous speech production data have been previously reported (Stenneken, Hofmann, & Jacobs, 2005c).

RESULTS

Phoneme analyses

The data set of KP's neologistic utterances comprised 1643 phonemic units, which corresponded to 38 different German phonemes (when distinguishing tense and lax vowels). All segments were part of the German phoneme inventory and their combinations conformed to German phonotactics. Phoneme frequency analyses compared the frequencies of occurrence for the phonemes in the aphasic data to phoneme frequencies in the normative data. The two data sets were highly correlated ($r = .91, p < .001$). Thus, phonemes with a high frequency in German tended to occur more frequently in the aphasic data and those with a low frequency in German tended to occur less frequently (Figure 1). In particular, the distributions suggested a numerical tendency to produce high-frequency phonemes in KP. When assigning German phoneme frequencies to logarithmic frequency classes (class 1 starting from 10,000 occurrences, 2 starting from 100,000, 3 starting from 1,000,000), only 3% of the phonemes produced by KP fell into the lowest frequency class. About 47% of the phonemes were in the medium frequency range, and 48% fell into the highest frequency class. In contrast, relatively fewer phonemes in the standard data belonged to the highest frequency class (18% in frequency class 1, 66% in class 2, and 15% in class 3).

Additionally, to address dual units of phonemes, correlation analyses were performed on biphoneme frequencies, i.e., the frequencies of occurrence for biphonemes in the neologistic data and biphoneme frequencies in the normative data. Again, results showed that the two data sets were highly correlated ($r = .36$, $p < .001$), pointing to preferred occurrences of high-frequency dual units of phonemes in the aphasic neologisms, when the biphonemes were of high frequency in the standard language.

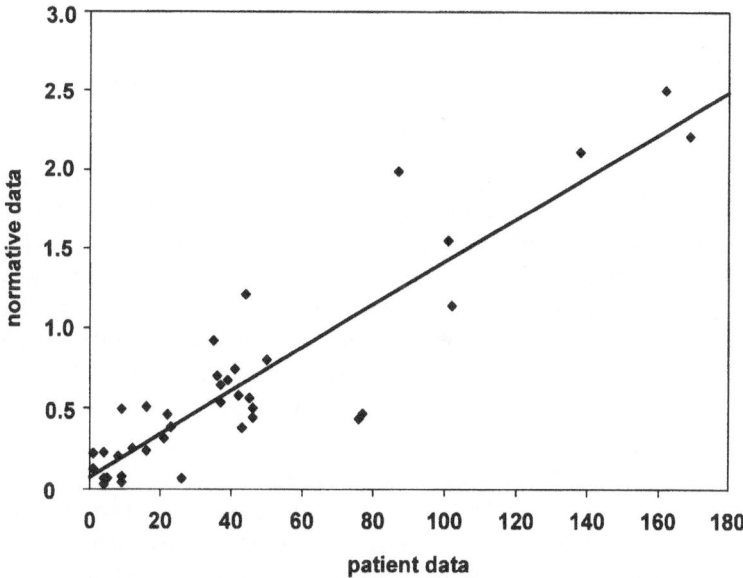

Figure 1. Scatterplot of phoneme frequencies in nonword errors of the aphasic jargon (patient data) and those in German (normative data: occurrences in millions).

Discussion. The present results showed that jargon-aphasic neologisms consisted of phonemes of the standard language and complied with its phonotactics. These findings from connected speech are in line with those of previous studies using a variety of language tasks (Buckingham & Kertesz, 1976; Butterworth, 1979; Christman, 1994; Duchan et al., 1980; Robson et al., 2003). Moreover, KP's neologisms showed a distribution of phoneme frequencies similar to that in the standard language. A comparable, though weaker, correlation was observed for biphonemes. In general, the findings point to a strong role of phonemic units in neologism formation. Comparable results for phoneme frequencies have been reported in one study of spontaneous speech utterances in an English-speaking jargon-aphasic patient (Hanlon & Edmondson, 1996). Other studies have shown an influence of phoneme frequency in jargon-aphasic naming errors (Robson et al., 2003) and in errors produced by aphasic patients without jargon in both spontaneous and structured speech tasks (Gordon, 2002). Together with the tendency in KP to produce high-frequency phonemes, the present findings suggest a strong influence from segmental phonology of the standard language on abstruse neologism generation. More specifically, phoneme inventory, phoneme combinations, and frequencies in KP point to undisturbed segmental phonology, even in jargon that does not show a clear influence of lexical targets or of neighbouring utterance units.

Syllable analyses

So far, analyses of aphasic neologisms focused on phonemic units, whereas little is known about the relevance of other sublexical units like syllables. The present analyses therefore compared the syllables in KP's neologisms to those of the standard language concerning the measures of syllable inventory, frequency distributions, and syllable structure. The data set of KP's neologisms comprised 600 syllabic units that corresponded to 310 different syllable types.

A comparison of the syllables in the aphasic data to the syllable inventory of the German database revealed that 47 of KP's syllables (corresponding to about 15% of the data) did not occur in the standard language, although all were phonologically legal. Further analyses determined the frequencies of occurrence for the syllables in KP's nonword errors and compared these to syllable token frequencies in the standard data. Results showed a significant positive correlation ($r = .600, p < .001$), indicating similar distributions of syllable frequencies in the two data sets (Figure 2). In addition, the distributional pattern pointed to a preferential use of high-frequency syllables in KP's neologisms. Logarithmic token frequency classes of syllables in the standard language were formed (i.e., occurrences of 10, 100, 1000, 10,000, and so on in German phonological word forms). In the neologism data, more syllables fell into higher logarithmic frequency classes. Results showed a continuous rise, with fewest syllables of KP (3%) belonging to the lowest frequency class, followed by 6%, 14%, 25%, 34% with increasing frequency classes. This observation did not extend to the highest logarithmic frequency class with only 9% of KP's syllables. However, this class of German syllables comprised only 11 different units, mostly representing monosyllabic function words. In contrast to the patient data, most German syllables belong to the lower frequency classes (35% to the lowest class, followed by 26%, 23%, and only 16% for all remaining high-frequency classes).

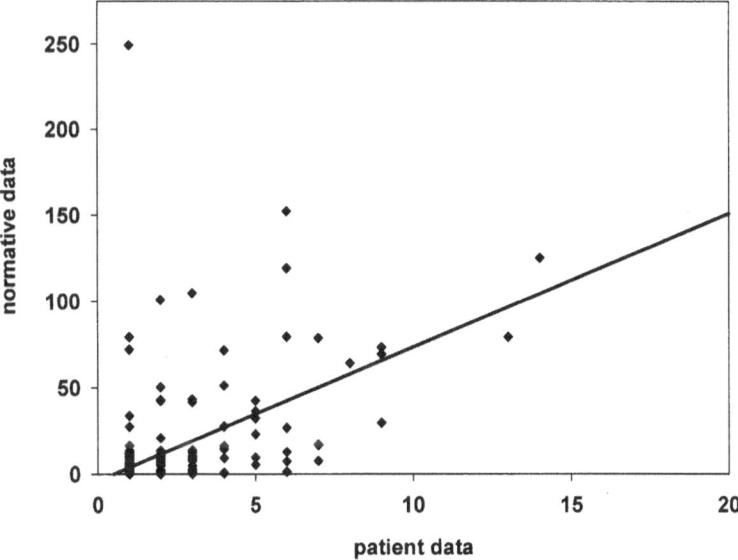

Figure 2. Scatterplot of syllable frequencies in nonword errors of the aphasic jargon (patient data) and those in German (normative data: occurrences in thousands).

As second syllabic measure, syllable complexity was determined for a data set of 277 syllables in KP's neologisms, which had been classified according to their sonority structures in previous analyses (Stenneken et al., 2005a). For the present purpose, the following complexity categories were derived for syllable onset and coda positions: no consonantal segments in onset or coda position (single vowel, V), single consonant in onset or coda (CV or VC), or clusters of two or three consonants (CCV or VCC, CCCV or VCCC). Clusters of more than three consonants made up only 0.5% of KP's data and therefore did not enter analyses. Results indicate that the distributions of syllable complexity types were also highly similar in the aphasic neologisms and in the standard language (Figure 3).

Discussion. The analyses of syllabic units have again revealed similarities between the aphasic neologisms and the standard language. These concerned the frequency distributions of syllables and syllable structures. Supported by a preferred use of high-frequency syllables in the aphasic neologisms, the present findings suggest a relevance of syllabic units in neologism formation.

One observation that seemed to contradict a linear relation of the two data sets may be discussed in more detail. The syllable /di/ has a rather low frequency in KP but an extraordinarily high frequency in standard German (about 250,000 occurrences; see Figure 2). This phonological unit not only occurs as a syllable in many German words but also corresponds to the feminine definite article (*die*) and thus also has a high word frequency. The observed results could therefore be due to the methodological procedure, in which identifiable real-word utterances in the patient data did not enter the analyses, leading to the exclusion of syllables that could also represent monosyllabic words. Thus this observation suggests—as has also been observed for phoneme frequencies—that the similarity in the distributions of the patient and the standard data express a general tendency but not a one-to-one equivalence in frequency ranks.

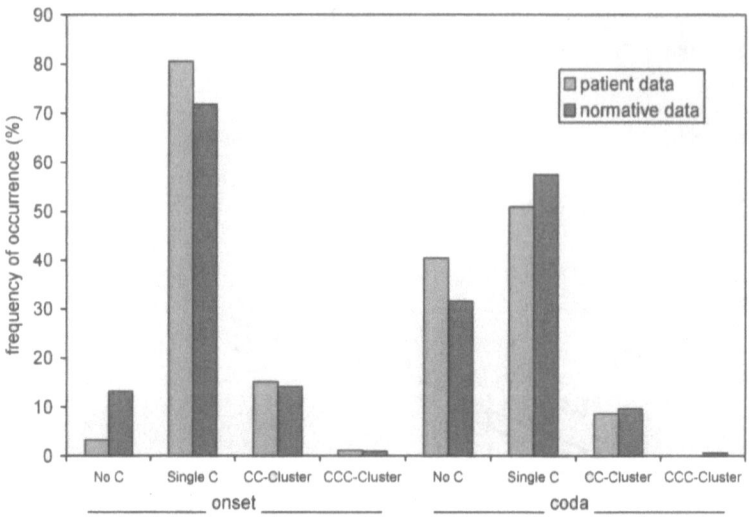

Figure 3. Distribution of syllable structures in nonword errors of the aphasic jargon (patient data) and in German (normative data) according to types of onset complexity (left side) and coda complexity (right side). (C = consonant in onset or coda positions, CC = double consonants, CCC = cluster of three consonants.)

Concerning syllable frequencies in aphasic neologisms, not much is known from previous studies. There is some evidence for syllable frequency effects from other language impairments, including aphasic patients with phonological production or reading deficits (Laganaro, 2005; Staiger, Ziegler, & Schmid, 2006; Stenneken, Conrad, Hutzler, Braun, & Jacobs, 2005b) or patients with apraxia of speech (Aichert & Ziegler, 2004a; Laganaro, 2008 this issue; Staiger & Ziegler, 2008 this issue). Here, the syllable frequency of target stimuli was shown to affect error rates or reaction times in a variety of tasks including repetition, reading aloud, visual lexical decision, and naming in German and French (but see Wilshire & Nespoulous, 2003, for null effects in two French-speaking aphasic patients). One of these studies (Staiger et al., 2006) focused on spontaneous speech productions and demonstrated that patients with aphasia showed a preferred use of high-frequency syllables in their spontaneous speech utterances.

The observations concerning syllable frequencies can be related to findings on syllable structures. The present results showed similar distributions of consonants in the syllable structures of aphasic neologisms and standard data. Consistent findings have been reported for sonority structures (Christman, 1992, 1994). Results indicated that syllabic sonority structures in non-target-related errors of jargon-aphasic patients conformed to the predictions for the standard language as derived from theory (Christman, 1992, based on Clements, 1990). Furthermore, when comparing target-related errors to their intended targets, the aphasic utterances showed either unchanged or decreased syllable complexity concerning the sonority profiles (Christman, 1994; for a similar tendency to theoretically preferred sonority profiles in connected speech, see previous analyses of KP in Stenneken et al., 2005a). Supportive evidence for a role of syllable structures, constrained by preferred sonority contours, in speech production comes from aphasia syndromes without jargon (Bastiaanse, Gilbers, & van der Linde, 1994; Den Ouden, 2002; Romani & Calabrese, 1998).

Based on the empirical findings of syllable frequency effects, it has been discussed whether phonological processing involves the retrieval of syllable-sized representations (Cholin, 2008 this issue; Conrad, Stenneken, & Jacobs, 2006; Laganaro & Alario, 2006). Although the results of the present study point to syllables as relevant processing units, the interpretation may be limited by the finding that, in the speech sample of patient KP, 15% of the syllabic units, all legal phoneme combinations like [tsɔm] or [lɛçt], did not occur as syllables in the standard language database. This observation argues against the assumption that KP's nonword errors are generated from chains of syllabic units, as has been suggested in a related way for phonemic units in abstruse neologism formation (cf. Buckingham, 1990). Rather, the finding of new-formed syllables would be compatible with the assumption that syllabic representations influenced other sublexical (e.g., segmental) processing domains. Supportive empirical evidence for an influence of other phonological processing domains on segmental processing comes from a patient with phonological jargon (Janßen & Domahs, 2008 this issue). Here, error analyses indicated that segmental processing was influenced by metrical processing. In the following section the different sublexical processing domains and their possible contributions will be further explored by additional analyses.

Regression analyses

A multiple linear regression analysis was conducted that took different sublexical measures into account. It explored whether a sublexical unit in the standard language can be identified that best predicts the frequency of occurrence for the aphasic nonword errors. The frequency of occurrence of KP's neologistic syllables served as criterion variable, and sublexical predictor variables were phoneme frequency, biphoneme frequency, and syllable frequency in the standard language. For each utterance unit in the patient data, the corresponding sublexical measures in the standard language were computed from the German word form database (Baayen et al., 1995) as syllable frequencies and as averaged frequencies for all phonemes or biphonemes occurring in the aphasic utterances. Since no word boundaries could be determined in the neologistic jargon, utterances were separated into syllabic units for the present analyses. The data set comprised 305 syllabic units in KP's neologisms, having excluded five units that consisted of a single vowel so that biphoneme frequencies could not be computed.

A significant model emerged, $F(3, 301) = 58.56$, $p < .001$; adjusted $R^2 = .362$. Results were significant only for syllable frequency ($t = 10.70$, $p < .001$), whereas biphoneme and phoneme frequency were not a significant predictor in this model (biphoneme frequency: $t = 1.40$, $p = .164$; phoneme frequency: $t = 0.29$, $p = .772$). With regard to the method of computing the different sublexical measures, these cannot be assumed to be completely independent of other. Additional analyses revealed a low correlation of syllable frequency and phoneme frequency ($r = .18$, $p < .001$), whereas syllable frequency and biphoneme frequency were moderately correlated ($r = .47$, $p < .001$).

Discussion. The results from regression analysis suggest that the averaged frequencies of phonemes and biphonemes, and the frequencies of syllables in the standard language, did not each contribute independently to the frequency of occurrence of KP's neologistic utterances; rather, only syllable frequency served as predictor for the frequency pattern of the aphasic utterances. Syllable frequency accounted for around 36% of the variance in the frequency of occurrence of the neologistic utterances. This finding, that syllable frequency is the factor that is crucially responsible for the variance in the aphasic data, supports a role of syllabic units in neologism formation. The present analyses did not include syllable structures, since these did not contain segmental information. Still, as stated above, the observed effect of syllable frequency would also be compatible with a relevance of syllables' structural information, since syllables with a higher frequency of occurrence also tend to have less complex syllable structures.

Moreover, the assumption of a prominent role of syllabic units does not contradict the observed similarities in phoneme frequency distributions for the aphasic and the normative data. Again, a correlation between the measures of phoneme and syllable frequencies would be expected, since a high frequency of occurrence for larger units, like words or syllables, is also reflected in a high frequency of constituent units, like phonemes. In general, it is hard to disentangle phoneme (or biphoneme) and syllable frequency effects. When a given utterance is segmented into phonemes, more observations are available than when the same utterance is segmented into syllables. In multiple regression analyses using phoneme and syllable frequency predictors, phoneme frequencies were averaged, whereas syllable frequencies were entered without prior transformation.[2] In general, the present methodological considerations point to the relevance of addressing different sublexical measures in the analyses of aphasic data (see Aichert & Ziegler, 2005; Hofmann, et al., 2007). To summarise, the present data seem to be best explained by assuming a prominent role of syllabic units in neologism formation. In the following section this interpretation will be discussed in more detail and related to the underlying deficit in KP.

GENERAL DISCUSSION

The present study revealed similarities in aphasic neologisms and the standard language for different sublexical measures. The results of the comparative analyses can be interpreted as follows: (1) Undisturbed segmental phonology can be assumed even for neologisms in which lexical influence is minimised. (2) Sublexical information, based on representations of syllabic units or structures of the standard language, seems to influence neologism formation.

With regard to the first assumption, evidence was provided by the phoneme inventory and the compliance with German phonotactics in the patient's neologisms. In addition, phonological processing in KP seemed to reflect the standard language's phoneme frequencies, in that phonemes of high frequency in German had a higher chance of being produced in the neologisms than those of lower frequencies. The present study extended previous evidence from English-speaking patients (e.g., Hanlon & Edmondson, 1996) for intact phonological processes in jargon aphasia by findings from an additional phonology, German, that allows for rather complex

---

[2] Comparable findings were obtained in regression analyses that alternatively employed the *minima* of phoneme, biphoneme, and syllable frequencies, $F(3, 301) = 59.66$, $p < .001$; adjusted $R^2 = .367$. Results still indicated that syllable frequency was the best predictor ($t = 7.23$, $p < .001$). In addition, the results were significant for biphoneme frequency ($t = 2.09$, $p = .038$); however, this measure might not have a strong individual contribution as it appeared to be highly correlated with syllable frequency ($r = .74$, $p < .001$).

phonological structures. In sum, results from phoneme analyses supported the notion that phonemes are functionally relevant production units in neologism formation. In addition to most previous phonological investigations of aphasic nonword errors, the present study also demonstrated phonemic similarities for utterances in which lexical influence can be assumed to be minimised. The assumption of a lexical impairment in KP was confirmed by several aspects in his language production. In connected speech, hardly any phonemic paraphasias were observed that would have pointed to a phonemic distortion of lexical targets. Neologisms were embedded in passages of intelligible speech and tend to occur in slots in which a content word would be expected, compatible with the notion of neologisms as surrogate forms in case of impaired lexical access. Similarly, in structured language tasks, there was no clear evidence for a phonemic relatedness of KP's responses to their targets (Stenneken et al., 2005a). In general, neologisms were variable in their phonological form and inconsistent responses are made to identical items, arguing against a deficient lexical representation. In sum, this pattern in the speech production of KP would be compatible with the association of neologism formation to impaired lexical retrieval or lost phonological information (cf. Buckingham & Kertesz, 1976; Butterworth, 1979) and the implication that segmental phonology would proceed disconnected from lexical processing (Hanlon & Edmondson, 1996).

An alternative interpretation of KP's disorder would be to assume a lexical origin of the neologism formation, in which word forms are phonemically distorted after lexical selection. Here, lexical selection can either be assumed to be unimpaired or to involve errors in selecting the wrong form (discussion in Robson et al., 2003). Since phoneme frequency is marked not only at the phoneme but also on the lexical level, the observed similarities in the neologism to the standard language might also reflect the phonemic structure of a lexical target. On the basis of the present data, this interpretation cannot be excluded as the source of KP's neologism generation. However, with regard to completely incomprehensible neologistic utterances, a severe distortion of the phonological form of the lexical item must be assumed, so that the target's phonemic structure is not evident from the neologistic utterance. It is not possible to finally decide between these two alternative accounts of neologism formation—both would allow for the conclusion that the observed similarity of the aphasic errors to the standard language could hardly be attributed to the phonemic content of a certain lexical target.

The second, novel aspect of the present investigations regarded the role of syllabic units in neologism formation. So far, evidence for undisturbed sublexical processing mainly concerned segmental phonological processing. The present findings indicated that syllable frequencies are also distributed similarly in neologisms and in standard German. Moreover, a strong relevance of syllables in neologism generation was suggested by the effects of syllable frequency, i.e., finding that syllable frequency in the standard data served as the predictor of the frequencies of the jargon-aphasic utterances.

On the one hand, the present findings would be compatible with the assumption that syllables are individually represented and retrieved in speech production. A specific view has been proposed by the concept of the syllabary, from which gestural scores for high-frequency syllables are assumed to be accessed during phonetic encoding (Levelt, Roelofs, & Meyer, 1999; Levelt & Wheeldon, 1994). On the other hand, the interpretation is restricted by an observation concerning syllable types. As discussed above, the finding of 15% new-formed syllables in the aphasic neologisms makes it unlikely that neologisms are composed as chains of syllabic units from the standard language. Rather, the findings from syllable structure and syllable complexity allow for an alternative view, according to which the observed effect of syllable frequency might result from structural syllable computation. Assuming a preference for non-complex syllables, the emerging utterances should also show a tendency for higher-frequent syllables. In more general terms, syllabic representations might play a role in neologism formation in that it constrains processing in other sublexical domains. The observation that the phonemic sequences in KP deviated from those of lexical forms can be related to the notion of an *indexing failure* while accessing the syllable nodes, which has been suggested to underlie speech errors in normal language production (Levelt et al., 1999; for a related account of segmental errors in an aphasic speaker, see Aichert & Ziegler, 2004b).

Moreover, the above considerations are compatible with models of speech production that assume an explicit representation of the structural information of syllables (cf. Dell, 1988; Shattuck-Hufnagel, 1992). This framework, in contrast to models that assume access to represented syllabic units or gestures, has been directly related to neologism production in aphasia (Dell et al., 1997; Hillis et al., 1999, Robson et al., 2003). It has been proposed that neologisms arise from a global weakening of connections in the model's connectionist architecture (Schwartz, Saffran, Bloch, & Dell, 1994) or from a local impairment of the connections between the lexical and the phonological level (Hillis et al., 1999). Both views would predict a reduced influence from the lexical level on the phonological nodes, which would facilitate the selection of non-target segmental information. Moreover, this type of model can account well for an additional observation in the present study, i.e., the tendency of KP's neologisms to include high-frequency sublexical units. Assuming that phonemes or syllable structures with high frequency in the standard language need less activation to reach the selection threshold as compared to units of lower frequencies, the model would predict a stronger tendency to produce high-frequency units the weaker the influence from the lexical nodes.

In general, the present study suggested that neologism generation is determined by sublexical characteristics of the standard language, even for connected jargonised speech that does not allow identification of lexical targets. More specifically, results point to a prominent role of syllabic representations that are unaffected by a lexical impairment and may influence segmental processing in neologism generation. Finally, findings from both phoneme and syllable analyses are compatible with an increased relevance of the standard language's sublexical principles when lexical influences are minimised.

REFERENCES

Aichert, I., & Ziegler, W. (2004a). Syllable frequency and syllable structure in apraxia of speech. *Brain and Language, 88,* 148–159.

Aichert, I., & Ziegler, W. (2004b). Segmental and metrical encoding in aphasia: Two case reports. *Aphasiology, 18,* 1201–1211.

Aichert, I., & Ziegler, W. (2005). Is there a need to control for sublexical frequencies? *Brain and Language, 95,* 170–171.

Baayen, R. H., Piepenbrock, R., & Gulikers, L. (1995). *The CELEX lexical database* [CD-ROM]. Philadelphia: Linguistic Data Consortium, University of Pennsylvania.

Bastiaanse, R., Gilbers, D., & van der Linde, K. (1994). Sonority substitutions in Broca's and conduction aphasia. *Journal of Neurolinguistics, 8*, 247–255.

Buckingham, H. W. (1990). Abstruse neologisms, retrieval deficits and the random generator. *Journal of Neurolinguistics, 5*, 215–235.

Buckingham, H. W., & Kertesz, A. (1976). *Neologistic jargon aphasia.* Amsterdam: Swets & Zeitlinger.

Butterworth, B. (1979). Hesitation and the production of verbal paraphasias and neologisms in jargon aphasia. *Brain and Language, 8*, 133–161.

Butterworth, B. (1985). Jargon aphasia: Processes and strategies. In S. Newman & R. Epstein (Eds.), *Current perspectives in dysphasia* (pp. 321–352). Edinburgh, UK: Churchill Livingstone.

Cholin, J. (2008). The mental syllabary in speech production: An integration of different approaches and domains. *Aphasiology, 22*, 1127–1141.

Christman, S. S. (1992). Uncovering phonological regularity in neologisms: Contributions of sonority theory. *Clinical Linguistics and Phonetics, 6*, 219–247.

Christman, S. S. (1994). Target-related neologism formation in jargonaphasia. *Brain and Language, 46*, 109–128.

Clements, G. N. (1990). The role of sonority in core syllabification. In J. Kingston & M. E. Beckman (Eds.), *Papers in laboratory phonology I. Between the grammar and physics of speech* (pp. 283–333). Cambridge, UK: Cambridge University Press.

Conrad, M., Stenneken, P., & Jacobs, A. M. (2006). Associated or dissociated effects of syllable frequency in lexical decision and naming. *Psychonomic Bulletin & Review, 13*, 339–345.

Dell, G. S. (1988). The retrieval of phonological forms in production: Tests of predictions from a connectionist model. *Journal of Memory and Language, 27*, 124–142.

Dell, G. S., Schwartz, M. F., Martin, N., Saffran, E. M., & Gagnon, D. A. (1997). Lexical access in aphasic and nonaphasic speakers. *Psychological Review, 104*, 801–838.

den Ouden, D. B. (2002). Segmental vs syllable markedness: Deletion errors in the paraphasias of fluent and non-fluent aphasics. In E. Fava (Ed.), *Clinical linguistics: Theory and applications in speech pathology and therapy. Current issues in linguistic theory 227* (pp. 23–45). Amsterdam: John Benjamins.

Dogil, G., Hildebrandt, G., & Schürmeier, K. (1990). The communicative function of prosody in a semantic jargon aphasia. *Journal of Neurolinguistics, 5*, 353–369.

Duchan, J. F., Stengel, M. L., & Oliva, J. (1980). A dynamic model derived from the intonational analysis of a jargon aphasic patient. *Brain and Language, 9*, 289–297.

Gordon, J. K. (2002). Phonological neighborhood effects in aphasic speech errors: Spontaneous and structured contexts. *Brain and Language, 82*, 113–145.

Hanlon, R., & Edmondson, J. A. (1996). Disconnected phonology: A linguistic analysis of phonemic jargon aphasia. *Brain and Language, 55*, 199–212.

Hillis, A., Boatman, D., Hart, J., & Gordon, B. (1999). Making sense out of jargon: A neurolinguistic and computational account of jargon aphasia. *Neurology, 53*, 1813–1824.

Hofmann, M. J., Stenneken, P., Conrad, M., & Jacobs, A. M. (2007). Sublexical frequency measures for orthographic and phonological units in German. *Behavior Research Methods, 39*(3), 620–629.

Huber, W., Poeck, K., Weniger, D., & Willmes, K. (1983). *Aachener Aphasie Test.* Göttingen: Hogrefe.

Janßen, U., & Domahs, F. (2008). Going on with optimised feet: Evidence for the interaction between segmental and metrical structure in phonological encoding from a case of primary progressive aphasia. *Aphasiology, 22*, 1157–1175.

Kertesz, A., & Benson, D. (1970). Neologistic jargon: A clinicopathological study. *Cortex, 6*, 362–386.

Kohn, S., Smith, K., & Alexander, M. (1996). Differential recovery from impairment to the phonological lexicon. *Brain and Language, 52*, 129–149.

Laganaro, M. (2005). Syllable frequency effect in speech production: Evidence from aphasia. *Journal of Neurolinguistics, 18*, 221–235.

Laganaro, M. (2008). Is there a syllable frequency effect in aphasia or in apraxia of speech or both? *Aphasiology, 22*, 1191–1200.

Laganaro, M., & Alario, F.-X. (2006). On the locus of the syllable frequency effect in speech production. *Journal of Memory and Language, 55*, 178–196.

Lecours, A. R. (1982). On neologisms. In J. Mehler, S. Franck, E. Walker, & M. Garret (Eds.), *Perspectives of mental representation* (pp. 217–247). Hillsdale, NJ: Lawrence Erlbaum Associates Inc.

Levelt, W. J. M., Roelofs, A., & Meyer, A. S. (1999). A theory of lexical access in speech production. *Behavioral and Brain Sciences, 22*, 1–75.

Levelt, W. J. M., & Wheeldon, L. (1994). Do speakers have access to a mental syllabary? *Cognition, 50*, 239–269.

Marshall, J. (2006). Jargon aphasia. What have we learned? *Aphasiology, 20*, 387–410.

Perecman, E., & Brown, J. W. (1981). Phonemic jargon: A case report. In J. W. Brown (Ed.), *Jargonaphasia* (pp. 177–258). New York: Academic Press.

Peuser, G., & Temp, K. (1981). The evolution of jargon aphasia. In J. W. Brown (Ed.), *Jargonaphasia* (pp. 259–294). New York: Academic Press.

Robson, J., Pring, T., Marshall, J., & Chiat, S. (2003). Phoneme frequency effects in jargon aphasia: A phonological investigation of nonword errors. *Brain and Language, 85*, 109–124.

Romani, C., & Calabrese, A. (1998). Syllabic constraints in the phonological errors of an aphasic patient. *Brain and Language, 64*, 83–121.

Schwartz, M., Saffran, E., Bloch, D., & Dell, G. (1994). Disordered speech production in aphasic and normal speakers. *Brain and Language, 47*, 52–88.

Shattuck-Hufnagel, S. (1992). The role of word structure in segmental serial ordering. *Cognition, 42*, 213–259.

Staiger, A., & Ziegler, W. (2008). Syllable frequency and syllable structure in the spontaneous speech production of patients with apraxia of speech. *Aphasiology, 22*, 1201–1215.

Staiger, A., Ziegler, W., & Schmid, G. (2006). *Frequency and structure of sublexical units in the spontaneous speech production of apraxic and aphasic patients.* Presentation at the Science of Aphasia Meeting VII, Porto Conte, Italy.

Stenneken, P., Bastiaanse, R., Huber, W., & Jacobs, A. M. (2005a). Syllable structure and sonority in language inventory and aphasic neologisms. *Brain and Language, 95*, 280–292.

Stenneken, P., Conrad, M., Hutzler, F., Braun, M., & Jacobs, A. M. (2005b). Frequency effects with visual words and syllables in a dyslexic reader. *Behavioural Neurology, 16*, 103–117.

Stenneken, P., Hofmann, M., & Jacobs, A. M. (2005c). Patterns of phoneme and syllable frequency in jargon aphasia. *Brain and Language, 95*, 221–222.

Wilshire, C. E., & Nespoulous, J. L. (2003). Syllables as units in speech production: Data from aphasia. *Brain and Language, 84*, 424–447.

APHASIOLOGY, 2008, 22 (11), 1157–1175

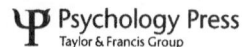

Going on with optimised feet: Evidence for the interaction between segmental and metrical structure in phonological encoding from a case of primary progressive aphasia

Ulrike Janßen

University of Marburg, Germany

Frank Domahs

University Clinic of the RWTH Aachen University, Germany

Background: Our knowledge about the interaction between segmental and metrical levels of representation in word production is still largely underspecified. In particular, there is only sparse evidence of how syllables are hierarchically organised into higher-level prosodic structures such as prosodic feet and words. Furthermore, the question whether stress assignment in German is sensitive to syllable weight is unresolved so far. While quantity-insensitive accounts state that stress is predominantly assigned to a default position (i.e., to the penultimate syllable) and other stress patterns are exceptional, quantity-sensitive accounts assume that stress assignment is determined by the weight of the final two syllables.

Aims: Impaired lexical retrieval may lead to regularisations of stress assignment. Such an error pattern will be examined to gain insights into the interrelation between different tiers of prosodic representations (e.g., syllable, foot, prosodic word).

Methods & Procedures: A reading and a repetition task were conducted with German-speaking patient HT, suffering from primary progressive aphasia, which especially affected her retrieval of lexical information. The material consisted of polysyllabic words with varying stress patterns and syllable structures.

Outcomes & Results: In reading, HT produced hardly any segmental errors, but a substantial amount of stress errors. Importantly, the patient not only over-generalised the "default" penultimate stress as would have been predicted by quantity-insensitive approaches. Instead, she over-applied different stress patterns depending on the weight of the last two syllables. In repetition, HT's output can be characterised as phonological jargon. Crucially, however, she hardly produced any stress errors. Rather, thorough analyses revealed that segmental deviations in her output led to optimised prosodic structures. For instance, insertions of rhyme segments could be observed mainly in strong syllables, i.e., syllables bearing main or secondary stress, whereas deletions occurred predominantly in weak, unstressed syllables.

Conclusions: The present data provide evidence for specific forms of interaction between segmental and metrical knowledge: On the one hand, segmental information influenced the patient's stress assignment errors in reading. On the other hand, prosodic

Address correspondence to: Ulrike Janßen, Institute for Germanic Linguistics, University of Marburg, Wilhelm-Roepke-Strasse 6a, 35032 Marburg, Germany. E-mail: janssenu@staff.uni-marburg.de

The present investigation was supported by the German Science Foundation (project WI 853/7-1) and by the START programme of the faculty of Medicine at the RWTH Aachen University (AZ 37/07). We would like to thank patient HT for participating in our studies, Anna-Lisa Schelwies for her assistance in transcribing some of the data, and Ingrid Aichert for kindly providing us with syllable frequency counts.

DOI: 10.1080/02687030701820436

information modified segmental errors even in severe jargon observed in repetition. With respect to the prosodic system of German, the observed error patterns show that the structure of the final syllable determines how syllables of a word are parsed into prosodic feet and, accordingly, which syllable has to be prominent. Thus, our results support quantity-sensitive approaches of stress assignment.

Keywords: Word stress; Prosody; Regularisation; Reading; Repetition.

INTRODUCTION

Impairments of phonological encoding are a widely observed symptom in aphasic speech production. In most cases phonologically deviant utterances have been attributed to difficulties in the selection and concatenation of segments to build syllables and phonological words (for an overview see Nickels, 1997). However, some observations also point to an interaction between such segmental errors and the metrical structure of affected words. First, data from aphasia as well as from language acquisition have repeatedly shown that segmental errors are more likely to occur in unstressed syllables (including schwa syllables), whereas stressed syllables are typically more preserved (Howard & Smith, 2002; Nickels & Howard, 1999; Niemi, Koivuselka-Sallinen, & Hanninen, 1985). Furthermore, Nickels and Howard (1999) as well as Howard and Smith (2002) found that patients suffering from phonological impairments produced significantly more omission and substitution errors in words consisting of a weak–strong pattern (e.g., *canóe*) compared to words with a strong–weak pattern (e.g., *rómance*).

With respect to errors affecting the metrical structure of a target, a study reported by Aichert and Ziegler (2004a) described a patient (WK) who tended to turn monosyllabic words into bisyllabic trochaic words (i.e., words consisting of a strong followed by a weak syllable). Furthermore, case studies reporting English- and Italian-speaking patients with surface dyslexia (Cappa, Nespor, Ielasi, & Miozzo, 1997; Gallante, Tralli, Zuffi, & Avanzi, 2000; Laganaro, Vacheresse, & Frauenfelder, 2002; Marshall & Newcombe, 1973; Miceli & Caramazza, 1993) have shown that such patients produced not only segmental but also suprasegmental regularisation errors (e.g., English: *bégin* instead of *begín*; Italian: *numíro* instead of *número*). In all these studies regularisation meant the over-generalisation of the most frequent or default stress pattern. For instance, Laganaro et al. (2002) described an Italian-speaking patient who produced stress errors in repetition as well as in reading and naming. Nearly all of his errors (93%) occurred in targets with "irregular" antepenultimate stress pattern

In sum, there is convincing evidence that segmental errors tend to be more likely in unstressed compared to stressed syllables and in words with an infrequent stress pattern. Thus, an influence of prosodic structure on segmental errors has been demonstrated, whereas the standard finding for metrical errors is that they follow the dominant pattern of the target language. Yet so far there are no reports describing the likelihood of prosodic errors being influenced by a word's segmental structure.

Moreover, up to now there are hardly any studies that have investigated segmental and suprasegmental errors in words longer than two syllables. Howard and Smith (2002) analysed phonological errors in trisyllabic words and found more errors in words with penultimate stress than in words with final or antepenultimate stress. This somewhat surprising observation indicates that postulating penultimate stress as the only unmarked stress pattern is unwarranted and needs further clarification.

Although in German—as in other Germanic languages—most native words are mono- or bisyllabic, the investigation of words longer than two syllables seems more appropriate to examine the influence of prosodic structure on phonological deficits. On the one hand, bisyllabic words often end in a schwa syllable, which cannot bear stress and, accordingly, these words do not provide alternative main stress positions. On the other hand, the investigation of longer words is capable of reflecting the whole prosodic system with its unmarked and marked foot structures and stress patterns, since main stress might occur on one of the three final syllables. In particular, it can be tested whether stress patterns are determined by the weight of syllables as has been proposed by some approaches on German stress assignment (see below).

Prosodic rosodic structure of german words

According to theories on metrical stress (Giegerich, 1985; Hayes, 1995; Kager, 1989; Liberman & Prince, 1977), stress is a relation between prominent and weak syllables that is realised via phonetic parameters such as fundamental frequency (F_0), duration, and intensity. The relational property of stress can be expressed on the basis of metrical feet, which assign strong and weak syllables to metrical patterns, for instance a strong and a weak syllable to a trochaic foot (e.g., *Tángo*, "tango") or a heavy syllable (e.g., *Stadt*, "city") to a monosyllabic foot. All in all, the prosodic structure of words consists of two levels of hierarchy: (i) strong and weak syllables are parsed into feet (e.g., [taŋ$_s$go$_w$]) and (ii) strong and weak feet are parsed into prosodic words (e.g., [oɐ.ga]$_w$[nɪs.mʊs]$_s$ "organism"). In German, only one of the final three syllables may bear stress ("three syllable window"; Giegerich, 1995; Wiese, 1996).

Some phonologists further propose that most stress positions in German words can be derived on the basis of syllable structure (e.g., Féry, 1998; Giegerich, 1985). According to such quantity-sensitive accounts, the final syllable of a word is stressed in words with a heavy(= closed) final syllable, and the prefinal syllable in words with a light(= open) final syllable. Regarding the occurrence of antepenultimate stress, theoretical explanations are controversial: Féry (1998) argues that antepenultimate stress occurs only in words with prefinal Schwa syllables (e.g., /ˈzɛ-[l]ə-ʁɪ:/ "celery"), whereas according to Giegerich (1985) it occurs in words with two light final syllables (e.g., [ˈaˑli-bi:] / ("alibi"). Janßen (2003a) provided experimental evidence for the assumption that the stress pattern in German words can be predicted to some extent from the structure of the final syllable: In a pseudoword reading task, words with a closed final syllable were mainly stressed on the final or antepenultimate syllable, while words with an open final syllable were predominantly stressed on the penultimate syllable.

However, quantity-sensitive accounts of German word stress are a challenge to proposals which claim that German has only one unmarked stress pattern, the final trochee, whereas final and antepenultimate stress patterns are marked and have to be specified in the lexical entry of a word (Eisenberg, 1991; Kaltenbacher, 1994; Levelt, Roelofs, & Meyer, 1999; Wiese, 1996). From a psycholinguistic perspective, Levelt et al. (1999) and Levelt (1999) propose in their model of word production that the metrical frame of words in most Germanic languages is filled from left to right and that the first syllable within a word containing a full vowel carries main stress. Such a metrical frame is said to be the default stress pattern, which is not lexically prespecified. The metrical information, which is part of the phonological representation of a word and thus retrieved during phonological encoding, consists of information about the number of syllables and the position of the strong syllable that has to bear the main stress within a word. According to this view, the latter type of information is stored for words with irregular stress only. The advantage of this model is to minimise the number of lexical specifications for languages that are predominantly stressed on the first syllable (e.g., German, Dutch, or English). However, Levelt et al.'s (1999) model is under-specified with respect to the hierarchy between syllables of a word, since their model specifies only the number of syllables and the position of main stress. Yet an analysis of prosodic structures of words consisting of three and more syllables revealed not only a twofold distinction between stressed and unstressed syllables, but also a threefold gradation between syllables with primary stress, secondary stress, and no stress at all (Alber 1997, 1998; see also Figure 1 for an illustration of such an analysis). Thus, it can be assumed that syllables are hierarchically structured within a word in terms of metrical feet. Such a gradation of prominence is also adopted in Gerken's (1996) *prosodic hierarchy hypothesis*, according to which the vulnerability of a syllable in child language depends on the integration of the syllable within the prosodic structure of a word. For instance, weak syllables embedded in a foot structure $(\sigma_S\ \sigma_W)_F$ are less prone to omission than unparsed weak syllables $(\sigma_W\ (\sigma_S\ \sigma_W)_F)$.

The present study

In the present study the interaction of segmental and metrical information in phonological encoding is examined in a patient who showed disorders of phonological encoding in the light of impaired lexical knowledge. It is assumed that impairments of lexical knowledge lead to the application of rules, such that errors reflect these rules as regularisations. The use of polysyllabic words with different metrical structure allows examination of the whole spectrum of possible metrical errors. For example, only the presentation of (at least) four-syllable words allows assessment of whether ill-formed utterances respect the three-syllable window of German. Two possible aspects of interaction are examined: (i) segmental information influencing metrical errors and (ii) metrical information influencing segmental errors.

First, the influence of segmental structure on metrical errors has not been reported so far. Yet specific predictions can be derived from quantity-sensitive accounts of stress assignment: If segmental structure remains unchanged, an optimisation of structure should lead to wrong assignment of penultimate stress predominantly in words with an open final syllable, while ultimate and antepenultimate stress should be over-applied mainly in targets with a closed final syllable. Second, although there is already some evidence for an influence of metrical structure on segmental errors (see above), quantity-sensitive accounts of stress assignment make more specific predictions: It is expected that if metrical structure remains unchanged, an regularisation or optimisation of structure should lead to the addition of rhyme consonants in stressed syllables, whereas in unstressed syllables rhyme consonants should be more likely to be omitted. Interestingly, both conditions—preserved segments in the light of stress errors and vice versa—are found within one single patient, although in two different tasks: reading and repetition.

a)   bisyllabic words

<u>penultimate</u>   <u>ultimate stress</u>

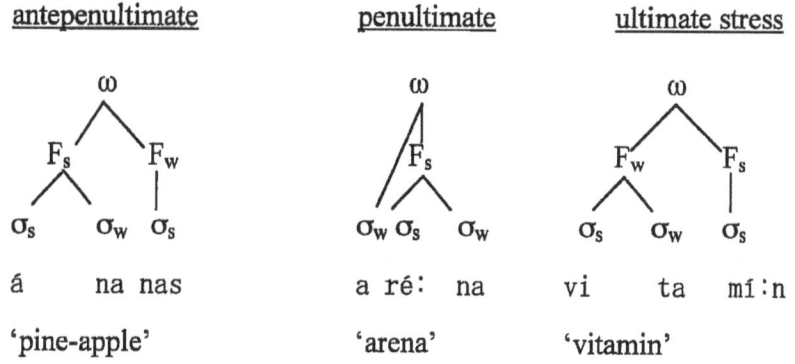

b)   trisyllabic words

<u>antepenultimate</u>   <u>penultimate</u>   <u>ultimate stress</u>

c)   quadrisyllabic words

<u>antepenultimate</u>   <u>penultimate</u>   <u>ultimate stress</u>

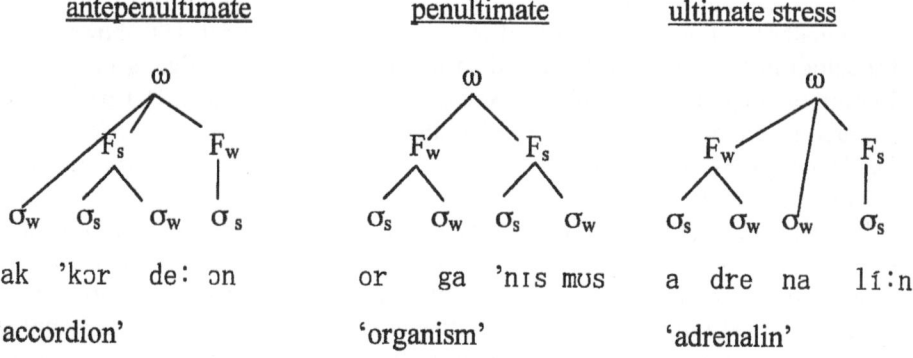

Figure 1. Metrical templates underlying phonological words with different stress pattern and syllable number (adopted from Alber 1997, 1998; Hayes 1995). Note that in words with final and antepenultimate stress, exhaustive parsing occurs only if they contain an odd number of syllables; in words with penultimate stress only if they contain an even number of syllables.

It becomes obvious that the investigation of interactions between segmental and metrical information as sketched so far may also be able to further constrain theories on metrical representation in general and stress assignment in particular. Specifically, the present study will try to provide evidence for a metrical structure similar to that assumed by Alber (1997, 1998) and Gerken (1996). Furthermore, the present investigation will address the question of whether stress assignment in German is quantity sensitive or not.

CASE DESCRIPTION

Patient HT, a right-handed housewife, was a native speaker of German with 8 years of formal education. At the time of our examination she was 56 years old. The patient's disorder was classified as *primary progressive aphasia* (PPA) according to the criteria of Mesulam (2001, p. 426). Her case was recently described in detail by Domahs, Bartha, Lochy, Benke, and Delazer (2006) with another focus of investigation. Some relevant background information will be repeated in the following.

HT first noticed problems in word finding 3 years before PPA was diagnosed. After that, her deficits became increasingly severe, albeit exclusively verbal in nature. Neuroradiological examinations revealed bilateral asymmetrical focal atrophy in the temporal lobes, affecting mainly lateral and inferior temporal areas (CT, MRI), and a loss of cortical and subcortical perfusion in the left temporal lobe (SPECT).

The patient showed a dramatically reduced working memory span for verbal material (digits: 2/1, letters: 1/2, months: 0/0 forward/backward, respectively) and a severely impaired verbal learning and memory performance. In contrast, her visual working memory (e.g., block tapping), visual perception and memory (e.g., Rey Osterreith Complex Figure; Osterreith, 1944; Rey 1941) and non-verbal reasoning (e.g., VESPAR; Langdon & Warrington, 1995) were largely intact. She showed no signs of apraxia.

The *Aachener Aphasie Test* (AAT; Huber, Poeck, Weniger, & Willmes, 1983) revealed compromised repetition (92/150 points), reading (25/30), and spelling (30/60) as well as poor comprehension (72/120) and a naming performance near floor (27/120). Her spontaneous speech was generally fluent with only a few phonological or syntactic errors. However, it consisted mainly of stereotypes bare of any recognisable content. Thus, in general HT's verbal processing was found to be severely impaired.

More specifically, Domahs et al. (2006) argued that the patient's deficit was functionally localised at the level of lexical processing. Indeed, HT showed severe difficulties in tasks that are assumed to test for lexical knowledge, such as lexical decision or assigning the gender-marked definite article to a noun. Her performance was modulated by word frequency and ambiguity, again pointing to a lexical locus of the deficit. Accordingly, her written language could be characterised as surface dysgraphia and surface dyslexia.

For example, a reading task of the *LeMo* battery (De Bleser, Stadie, Tabatabaie, & Cholewa, 2004, T 16) revealed that HT produced significantly more errors with irregular (61%) than with regular words (9%), indicating that HT had difficulties in retrieving lexical information. A qualitative error analysis, too, revealed symptoms of surface dyslexia, manifesting as regularisations of irregular forms—e.g., irregular *Garage* was realised as [ga'ra:gə] instead of /ga'ra:ʒə/.

Another observation important for the present investigation is that HT produced phonemic paraphasias in repetition tasks, as tested with the *AAT* subtest "word repetition" (92/150 points) and with subtests T 8 "non-word repetition" (28/40 correct) and T 9 "word repetition" (30/40) of the *LeMo* battery. Both a word frequency and a length effect became apparent. HT's errors were classified as substitutions, deletions, or insertions of segments.

READING TASK[1]

Given that the assignment of suprasegmental information to words is to some extent opaque in German, it must be lexically specified at least for a subset of words. Therefore, the breakdown of lexical knowledge in surface dyslexia might give us insights into the regularities of the German stress system. Following this logic, the present investigation aims to find out whether the segmental information of words modifies stress errors appearing in HT's surface dyslexic errors or vice versa. More specifically, we will examine whether the patient's regularisation errors are consistent with the predictions of quantity-sensitive accounts on German stress assignment (Féry, 1998; Giegerich, 1985; Janßen, 2003a). To address this question, we conducted a word-reading task with patient HT.

Method

Words with varying stress patterns and syllable structures were presented to HT. Since in German monomorphemic words stress is assigned to one of the final three syllables, we also used three- and four-syllabic words in addition to two-syllabic words. Altogether, 392 words were included in which each of the three possible stress positions occurred. The test material consisted of morphologically simple nouns only, in order to control for word category and complexity. Furthermore, the selected words varied with respect to the structure of their final and prefinal syllable (see Table 1 for an overview of stimulus conditions). Striving to present as many words as possible that fulfilled our criteria, we accepted a different number of items per condition.

Stimuli were presented visually in randomised order. The word list was printed in Arial typeface and 13 pt letter size. HT was asked to read aloud the words on the list. She was instructed to read the words as fluently as possible. If a word was read dysfluently, such that a prosodic analysis was made impossible, HT was encouraged to read the word again more fluently. The patient's responses were recorded and subsequently transcribed by three independent and phonetically trained listeners.

HT performed well in reading the target words fluently. After having read the stimulus, she always commented on whether she knew the meaning of that word or not. However, as a result of surface reading, HT had hardly ever access to the meanings of the stimuli presented. Of 392 stimuli, 7 (all quadrisyllabic words) were not analysable with respect to their stress pattern, because HT omitted syllables (e.g., [kas-ta:-ni:] instead of /kas-ta:-ni:-ə/), thus affecting the prosodic structure of the words. These words were excluded from analysis.

Results

Within the set of 385 analysable stimuli, HT produced 97 (25.2%) deviant stress patterns. In contrast, HT performed much better on the segmental level, as she made

---

[1] The reading task has been outlined very briefly in Janßen (2003b).

TABLE 1
Stimulus material for reading

Syllable number	Syllable structure		Stress pattern		
	Prefinal syllable	Final syllable	APU (N = 69) freq. 3.7	PU (N = 164) freq. 8.2	U (N = 152) freq. 10.6
σσ	open	open	-	10	4
(N = 93)	closed	open	-	11	1
	open	closed	-	17	17
	closed	closed	-	19	14
σσσ	open	open	25	31	12
(N = 252)	closed	open	3	31	1
	open	closed	26	13	79
	closed	closed	8	9	14
σσσσ	open	open	2	14	4
(N = 40)	closed	open	-	7	-
	open	closed	5	1	5
	closed	closed	-	1	1

Overview over the distribution of stress patterns in 385 analysable words that varied according to the number of syllables and the structure of the final and prefinal syllable. Open syllables end in a vowel and closed syllables end in a consonant. freq. = mean word frequencies per million according to the CELEX database (Baayen et al., 1995). APU = antepenultimate; PU = penultimate; U = ultimate stress.

only 10 segmental errors (2.6%; e.g., *Philosophie* read as [fi-lo-so-pi:] instead of /fi-lo-so-fi:/). Obviously, HT's surface reading manifested mainly in wrongly assigned stress patterns. However, in no single case did the patient violate the three-syllable window of German, i.e., she never assigned stress to the first syllable of a four-syllable word. As the accuracy scores depicted in Table 2 show, words with antepenultimate stress were more affected than words with penultimate or ultimate stress. Crucially, it was not the case that targets with penultimate stress—assumed to be the default pattern by proponents of quantity-insensitive accounts—were less error prone than targets with ultimate stress ("exceptions"). On the contrary, words with ultimate stress were least affected. Note that this cannot be due to a frequency advantage. Although Table 1 indicates that target words with ultimate stress were slightly more frequent than words with penultimate stress, this difference is not statistically significant (Mann-Whitney exact $p = .160$). Moreover, the mean frequency of *both* types of words can be considered as low (8.2 and 10.6 per million).

Table 3 presents examples of stress errors and the distribution of stress patterns involved in HT's suprasegmental errors. Interestingly, no instance of over-application of antepenultimate stress occurred, the pattern that was most error prone and which was replaced in 62.3% by either penultimate or ultimate stress. In

TABLE 2
Accuracy scores in reading for words with different stress patterns

	APU	PU	U
Total amount	26/69	120/163	142/153
Percentage correct	37.7%	73.6%	92.8%

APU = antepenultimate; PU = penultimate; U = ultimate stress.

TABLE 3
Examples of stress errors and distribution of involved stress patterns ("over-application") in reading

	Overapplication of	
Syllable number	penultimate stress	ultimate stress
σσ	/skan-dá:l/ → [skán-dal]	/mó:-nat/ → [mo-nát]
σσσ	/á-li-bi:/ → [a-lí-bi]	/kɛ-'ʁa:-mɪk/ → /kɛ-ʁa:-'mɪk/
σσσσ	/ha-mó-ni-ka/ → [ha-mo-ní-ka]	/ho-'mʊŋ-ku-lʊs/ → [ho-mʊŋ-ku-'lʊs]
Syllable structure		
open final	11/22 (50.0%)	23/134 (17.2%)
closed final	9/169 (5.3%)	54/99 (54.5%)
total	20/191 (10.5%)	77/233 (33.0%)

21% of these stress errors, penultimate stress was produced, and in 79% ultimate stress. Thus, penultimate stress was not the only pattern (over)used productively. This may be taken as further evidence that the final trochee is not the only regular stress pattern in German.

A closer look at the patient's stress errors revealed that her wrong assignment of stress was systematically related to the structure of the final syllable (Table 3, lower rows; Figure 2). Penultimate stress was over-generalised mainly to words with an open final syllable ($\chi^2 = 36.81$, $p < .01$), whereas ultimate stress was predominantly applied to words with a closed final syllable ($\chi^2 = 34.29$, $p < .01$).[2]

Overall, the data confirm theoretical assumptions (Féry, 1998; Giegerich, 1985) and empirical observations (Janßen, 2003a) on German stress assignment which state that the structural make-up of relevant (i.e., final) syllables has an impact on the placement of stress within a word.

REPETITION TASK

As shown above, segmental information, i.e., the presence or absence of a coda consonant in the final syllable, modified HT's stress errors in reading. In a subsequent word repetition task our aim was again to investigate the interaction between segmental and metrical tiers of information. Given her severe lexical impairment, we expected the patient to use a non-lexical processing route in repetition. In non-lexical repetition, regularisation may appear either as stress errors or as segmental errors. In the first case, similar patterns as observed in HT's reading may be produced. Indeed, Laganaro et al. (2002) described an Italian-speaking patient who produced similar stress errors in repetition, reading, and naming.

In the second case, segmental errors may be influenced by the metrical structure of the target word. For instance, prosodically prominent elements of speech (stressed syllables) can be expected to be less error prone than prosodically weaker elements (unstressed syllables) (Nickels & Howard, 1999; Niemi et al., 1985). Beyond this

---

[2] A pseudoword reading task also performed by HT revealed the same correlation between the structure of the final syllable and stress pattern: Pseudowords with a closed final syllable were stressed on the final syllable and pseudowords with an open final syllable on the prefinal syllable. Due to space limitations the pseudoword reading task will not be reported in more detail.

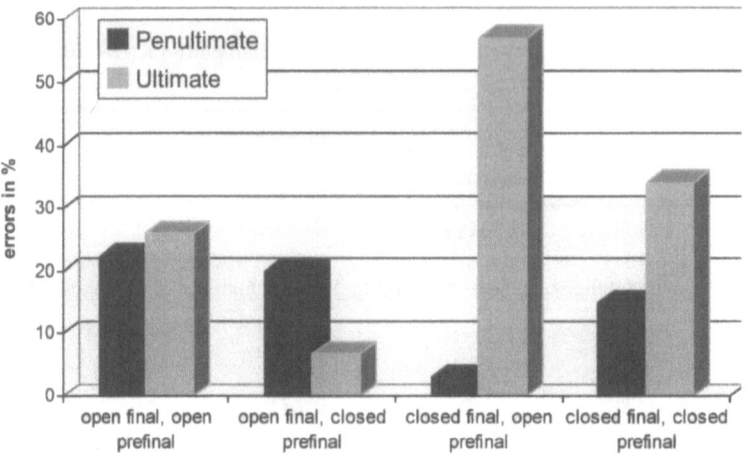

Figure 2. Distribution of wrong assignment of penultimate and ultimate stress in reading as a function of the target word's syllable structure. (HT never produced wrong antepenultimate stress.)

classic finding, however, quantity-sensitive approaches to stress assignment make more specific predictions. These predictions are related to the number as well as to the structure of syllables.

With respect to alterations in syllable number, i.e., deletion or insertion of a whole syllable, metrical theory predicts that unparsed syllables are particularly prone to be omitted (Gerken, 1996). Exhaustive parsing of syllables into feet is a crucial constraint on prosodic structure building in many languages, but may be violated if this leads to degenerate (i.e., incomplete) feet (Hayes, 1995). In language acquisition, Gerken (1996) found that weak syllables are especially prone to be omitted if they occurred in unparsed position (e.g., $ba_w[na_s.na_w]$) rather than in weak position within a foot (e.g., $[ti_s.ger_w]$). As can be seen in Figure 1, unparsed syllables occur (i) in words with penultimate stress containing an odd number of syllables or (ii) in words with ultimate or antepenultimate stress containing an even number of syllables. In these conditions deletion or addition of one syllable would lead to an optimised foot structure. Such an error pattern has not been investigated so far.

With respect to alterations in syllable structure, quantity-sensitive accounts predict that different kinds of errors should occur depending on the status of the affected syllable within prosodic structure. To be specific, segment *insertions* should appear mainly in strong (stressed) syllables, while segment *deletions* should predominantly affect weak (unstressed) syllables. Again, such an error pattern has not been described so far.

Method

Words from the same set as in the reading task were presented auditorily to HT. The stimuli were naturally spoken by a female German speaker, who was not informed about the purpose of the study to avoid exaggeration of the critical word information (prosodic strong vs weak positions). HT was asked to listen to each stimulus carefully and to repeat each word after its offset. During the repetition task, HT's responses were audio-taped and afterwards transcribed by three independent phonetically trained listeners. The repetition task was conducted in a separate session several weeks after the reading task. Therefore, possible interference between both tasks is assumed to be minimised.

Results

Out of the presented 322 stimuli only 201 responses could be considered in data analysis, since in the other cases HT either failed to repeat the presented word at all, or produced perseverations of preceding stimuli, or produced a wrong stress pattern, which happened only rarely (5 cases = 1.6%). Table 4 provides an overview over the distribution of stress pattern and syllable number in the remaining stimuli. HT's responses to the remaining 201 items revealed a severe impairment in word repetition with only 16% completely (i.e., segmentally as well as metrically) correct responses.

In the distorted utterances, substitutions, insertions, or deletions of segments led to the production of pseudowords with little phonological similarity to the target (phonological jargon). To investigate whether segmental errors were influenced by metrical structure, i.e., the structure of syllables, feet, and phonological words, data analysis was focused on insertions and deletions of segments because only such errors may affect the number and/or structure of syllables. Substitution errors were considered only in those cases in which a full vowel was replaced by a reduced vowel following the assumption that in such cases the vowel quality contributes to the syllable structure (Hayes, 1995; Kiparsky, 1979; Selkirk, 1982). Specifically, we analysed two types of segmental changes in more detail to examine the relationship between metrical structure and segmental errors: (a) deletions and insertions of syllables and (b) deletions/reductions and insertions of rhyme segments.

Changes in the number of syllables. A systematic analysis of 42 word repetition errors involving either an increase or a decrease in the number of syllables revealed that in 40 (95%) of these errors the main stress pattern of the target word was not affected by the change of syllable number. Only those 40 were entered into the data analysis. The number of syllables was changed by a maximum of 1. In responses with an increase in syllable number, in 24/31 (77%) cases HT inserted a syllable of the type Cə, where the C is mostly taken from the segmental material of the target word (16 cases, e.g., [ka-pə-'de:t] instead of /pa-'ke:t/ 'package'). Except for two insertions, the added material consisted of open syllables.

Crucially, insertions and deletions of syllables did not occur at random, but seemed to be guided by the stress pattern and the number of syllables of the target form. As

TABLE 4
Stimulus material for word repetition

Syllable number	Stress pattern		
	APU (N = 40)	PU (N = 75)	U (N = 86)
σσ (N = 39)	-	21	18
σσσ (N = 130)	33	38	59
σσσσ (N = 32)	7	16	9

Overview over the distribution of stress patterns in 201 analysable words varying according to the number of syllables. APU = antepenultimate; PU = penultimate; U = ultimate stress.

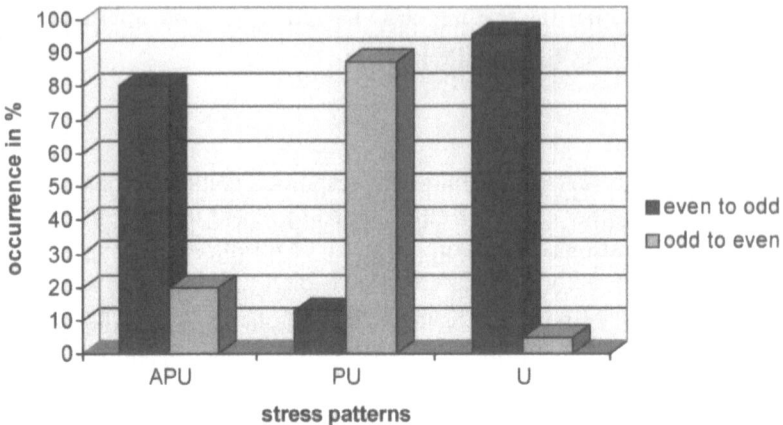

Figure 3. Direction of changes in syllable number in repetition as a function of the target word's stress pattern. Odd = 3 syllables; Even = 2 or 4 syllables. APU = antepenultimate; PU = ultimate; U = ultimate stress.

Figure 3 shows, some stress patterns seem to be systematically related to an even number of syllables, whereas other stress patterns are related to an odd number of syllables. In 12/38 (32%) trisyllabic words with penultimate stress, a syllable was inserted ([ma-[l]ə-'rɪ[l]ə] instead of /ma-'rɪ[l]ə/ 'apricot') and in one case a syllable was deleted (['ja:-tʊs] instead of /hi'ja:-tʊs/ 'hiatus'), both leading to a response with an even number of syllables. In target words with penultimate stress and an even number of syllables, only 2/37 (5.4%) additions (and no deletion) of a syllable were encountered (['ky-bə-rɪs] instead of /'kyɐ-bɪs/ 'pumpkin' and ['fɛ[m[əra] instead of /'fɪɐ-ma/ 'company'). Taken together, in words with penultimate stress 13/15 (86.7%) changes in syllable number resulted in nonwords with an even number of syllables. The dissociation between errors leading to an odd, and errors leading to an even, number of syllables was statistically significant ($\chi^2 = 7.90$; $p < .01$).

In contrast, changes of target words with either antepenultimate or ultimate stress led predominantly to a form with an odd number of syllables. For stimuli with antepenultimate stress, 4/7 (57%) quadrisyllabic words were realised as words containing five syllables (e.g., [ka-tsɪs-'za:-nɪ-jə] instead of /[kas-'ta:-nɪ-jə/ 'chestnut'). Such an addition error was observed only in 1/33 (3%) trisyllabic words (['kɛm-bə-la-də] instead of /'he:-ba[m]ə/ 'midwife'). A similar picture appeared for words with ultimate stress: In 11/18 (61%) bisyllabic words, HT added a light syllable which preceded the strong syllable (e.g., [ak-ze-'trat] instead of /aps-'trakt/ 'abstract') and in 8/9 (89%) quadrisyllabic words HT deleted a syllable (e.g., [kan-to-'li:n] instead of /ɪn-fan-tə-'ri:/ 'infantry'). Only in one case (1/59, 1.7%), a word with an odd number of syllables was turned into a word with an even number of syllables ([ke-ke-də'dɛns] instead of /ɛk-sɪs-'tɛns/ 'existence'). Taken together, errors involving a change in syllable number of target words with antepenultimate and ultimate stress led predominantly to an odd number of syllables. This dominance was statistically significant ($\chi^2 = 62.36$; $p < .001$).

Overall, the distribution of syllable insertions and deletions suggests that words with different stress patterns "prefer" different word templates in terms of syllable number (for a comparison see Figure 1).

Changes in syllable structure. In the present analyses we excluded all responses that entailed alterations of syllable *number*. We found 159 syllables within 126 words that were phonologically distorted due to deletion, insertion, or substitution of segments. These errors led to changes in syllable *structure* in 101 cases, which were included into analyses.

Overall, the data revealed that syllables bearing main stress were less error prone (16/101, 15.8%) than unstressed syllables or syllables with secondary stress (85/101, 84.2%). With respect to syllable structure errors in stressed syllables, 11/16 (69%) responses resulted in an increase of syllable weight (e.g., [pro-to-'gɔln] instead of /pro-to-'kɔl/, 'protocol'), while only the remaining 5 errors lead to decreased syllable weight (e.g., [a-pa:-tɛn] instead of /a-pa:t-mɛnt/ 'apartment'). In a one-sided binomial test this deviance from chance distribution approached statistical significance ($p \leqslant .067$).

A comparison of errors occurring in syllables with secondary stress and in weak syllables further indicates that additions or omissions of rhyme segments are related to the metrical prominence of a syllable. As can be seen in Figure 4, in syllables with secondary stress most errors consisted of *insertions* of rhyme segments (32/34 = 94%), while in unstressed syllables most errors were *reductions* of rhymes (45/51 = 88%). The majority of errors in syllables with secondary stress were instances of additions of coda consonants (31/32 = 97%, e.g., ['kɔ[l]ə-ral] instead of /'kɔ[l]ə-ra/ 'cholera'), whereas most reduction errors in unstressed syllables involved a change in vowel quality, i.e., full vowels were altered into the reduced vowel [ə] (37/45 = 82%, e.g., [ma-gə-'tsi:n] instead of /ma-ga-'tsi:n/ 'magazine'). Taken together, the observed error patterns clearly show that the type of segmental error (omission, insertion, or vowel change) depends on the metrical position of a syllable within the phonological word ($\chi^2 = 52.07$, $p < .001$).

GENERAL DISCUSSION

We conducted two tasks—word reading and repetition—with HT, a patient with a predominant lexical impairment due to primary progressive aphasia. HT's regularisation errors allowed us to examine the interaction between segmental and metrical information during phonological encoding. Interestingly, both tasks led to

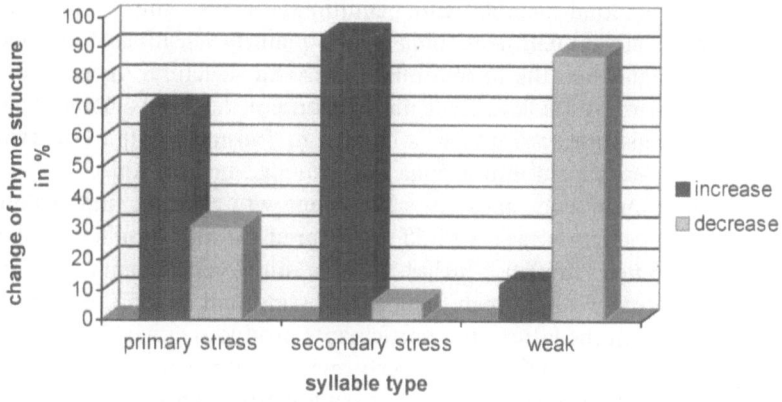

Figure 4. Type of segmental error in repetition as a function of syllable prominence. Increase/decrease refers to the change of syllable weight.

different patterns of errors: While in reading most errors affected the assignment of word stress, and segmental information remained largely unaffected, the opposite was true in repetition. In the light of HT's reduced memory span this dissociation between tasks may be explained by different task demands on working memory. In reading, segmental information may be repeatedly updated from orthographic information, whereas stress is not coded in German orthography. In repetition, however, no segmental update is possible, but it may be assumed that information about word stress and number of syllables can be memorised more easily than the segmental make-up of words, and may thus be less prone to memory decay. In the following, we will first discuss results from reading and then results from repetition.

Stress errors in reading

The reported data add to the evidence that patients with surface dyslexia not only produce segmental errors, but also deviant stress patterns (e.g., Marshall & Newcombe, 1973; Miceli & Caramazza, 1993). Indeed, most of HT's errors affected stress. Since surface reading is caused by impaired retrieval of word-specific lexical knowledge, one can assume that the observed errors are mostly regularisations of irregularly stressed words. The absence of lexical information during the reading task is further supported by the fact that HT was not able to access meaning of the words presented. Thus, HT's word reading performance is in some way comparable with pseudoword reading.

The distribution of her errors was not random. First, words with antepenultimate stress, a pattern that has been considered as irregular (Féry, 1998; Kaltenbacher, 1994), were particularly affected: out of the 73 targets with antepenultimate stress, 45 were realised with either penultimate or final stress. In no case was antepenultimate stress produced for targets with penultimate or ultimate stress. It seems very unlikely that this finding can be explained on the basis of segmental cues only.

However, concerning the stress patterns that were involved in wrong stress assignment, the data revealed that HT overused not just one default stress pattern to irregularly stressed words, as would be predicted by quantity-insensitive accounts on German word stress (Eisenberg, 1991; Kaltenbacher, 1994; Levelt et al., 1999). Rather, two patterns emerged, depending on the structure of the final syllable: Words with a closed final syllable were mainly realised with ultimate stress and words with an open final syllable with penultimate stress. This finding not only suggests that stress assignment is to some extent quantity sensitive. It also indicates that stress assignment, i.e., the formation of prosodic structure, operates from the right edge of the word to the left. First, the structure of the final syllable is checked. If it is heavy, it constitutes a foot on its own (e.g., $[bʊ-mə]_F[ráŋ]_F$). Otherwise, the two final syllables are parsed into a final trochee (e.g., $mɔs'[ki:-to]_F$).

Such a distribution of error patterns is consistent with previous findings obtained in a pseudoword production task with 25 unimpaired German adults who showed a comparable preference (Janßen, 2003a). In this study, participants used prefinal stress in 82% of words with an open final syllable, and only in 25% of words with a closed final syllable. In the latter case, participants produced either final stress (38%) or antepenultimate stress (37%). HT's performance with words is comparable to those of unimpaired participants with pseudowords, since she also avoided highlighting the prefinal syllable in words with a closed final syllable. However, for the group of unimpaired participants, the antepenultimate syllable was not a dispreferred stress position. In the present study, target words with antepenultimate stress were significantly less frequent than words with one of the other two stress patterns. Thus, a frequency-based explanation of the patient's particular deficit with words of the former type cannot be excluded. However, words of all conditions were of low frequency (see Table 1), somewhat weakening this argument. Another tentative interpretation for the dissociation between the use of antepenultimate stress by HT and by the healthy participants of Janßen (2003a) may be related to the direction of stress assignment: Most phonological theories agree that word stress in German is assigned starting from the right edge of a word (Eisenberg, 1991; Féry, 1998; Giegerich, 1985; Kaltenbacher, 1994; Wiese, 1996). Following this assumption, it seems plausible that stress assignment relies on increasing working memory resources in the following order: ultimate < penultimate < antepenultimate. If this is true, the patient's severely reduced working memory capacity may have caused a strong disadvantage for the production of antepenultimate stress.

In sum, surface dyslexic errors may provide evidence for unmarked prosodic patterns in a language. In the particular case of the German stress system, the present data have shown that German has not only one productive stress pattern but at least two—depending on the structure of the final syllable. More specifically, the presence or absence of a coda segment seems to be crucial for the metrical structure of a word.

Segmental errors in repetition

Segmental errors obtained in a word repetition task suggest that such errors can be prosodically driven. Focusing on either segment insertions or deletions, our major findings were that (i) changes of syllable number did mainly depend on the stress pattern and its underlying metrical structure, and (ii) an increase or decrease of rhyme complexity was systematically related to the metrical status of the respective syllable within a phonological word.

With respect to changes of metrical templates due to insertions or deletions of syllables, the present data confirm observations reported by Aichert and Ziegler (2004a) that phonological impairments may lead to the over-generalisation of an unmarked metrical pattern. As Aichert and Ziegler (2004a) suggest, their patient WK turned monosyllabic words into bisyllabic forms stressed on the penultimate syllable and thus displaying the statistically dominant trochaic pattern. We think that HT's utterances can be regarded as metrical optimisations as well, although her paraphasic responses did not generally lead to a trochaic pattern. A detailed scrutiny of alterations in syllable number in words with two, three, or four syllables revealed a correlation between the stress pattern of a target form on the one side and the number of syllables produced on the other. Changes of syllable number could be observed in words with penultimate stress, if the target consisted of three syllables with a metrical structure as depicted in Figure 1.

Targets with either final or antepenultimate stress were prone to a change in syllable number mainly in words with an even number of syllables. Note that words with final and antepenultimate stress exhibit in most cases a heavy final syllable, which constitutes a foot on its own (see also Janßen, 2003a). The metrical templates of different stress patterns, illustrated in Figure 1, make clear why words with different stress patterns may show different types of error. Since words with final and antepenultimate stress consist of a final monosyllabic foot, words with an odd number of syllables are preferred. Thus, all syllables can be exhaustively parsed into feet. In contrast, words with penultimate stress consist of a final trochee demanding that the phonological word consists of an even number of syllables, as an even number of syllables avoids an initial unparsed or "stray" syllable.[3] Overall, the observed alterations in syllable number suggest that the final foot of a phonological word determines its optimal prosodic structure. Most importantly, the data show that the trochaic pattern is not the only unmarked foot pattern in German, otherwise HT might have inserted a syllable in final position in targets with ultimate stress (such as [e-vi-dɛn-'tsə]). However, such errors did not occur. We argue instead that both a final trochee and a final monosyllabic foot are unmarked metrical patterns and the distribution depends on the structure of the final syllable. Furthermore, the patient's errors provide evidence that monosyllabic feet are bound to final word positions, since HT turned initial stray syllables either into trochees or deleted them. Crucially, it should be emphasised that HT's utterances avoided stress clashes as well as unparsed syllables, therefore most changes in syllable number can be viewed as optimisations of metrical structure: Responses with penultimate stress preferably consisted of an even number of syllables and words with final or antepenultimate stress of an odd number. Note that marked metrical patterns not only led to syllable omissions, but in 40% of all errors changing syllable number they resulted in insertions of a syllable. Such error patterns show that segmentally more complex structures may be metrically less marked.

Generally, the observed error patterns are in line with Gerken's prosodic hierarchy hypothesis (1996), which assumes that weak syllables, which are not dominated by a foot, are vulnerable to omission. Beyond that, the present data show that unparsed syllables or defective feet might also lead to an insertion of a syllable in order to create a proper foot. Furthermore, we assume that data reported by Howard and Smith (2002) can also be analysed along with our hypothesis that parsing of syllables into feet depends on the structure of the final syllable and the number of syllables. Comparable to our findings, Howard and Smith (2002) report a higher proportion of errors in trisyllabic words with penultimate stress than in trisyllables with antepenultimate and final stress in both picture-naming and repetition tasks. Words with antepenultimate and final stress were equally well preserved. However, these authors interpreted their finding as surprising, since they expected more errors to occur with strong–weak–weak (SWW) words than with weak–weak–strong (WWS) words. In SWW words it was hypothesised that the final weak syllable is unparsed and should therefore be omitted or prone to segmental substitution errors. If one assumes the same foot structure building for WWS and SWW words, as proposed in the present account, the data reported by Howard and Smith (2002) fit smoothly into our interpretation that trisyllabic words with penultimate stress are more marked than trisyllables with final or antepenultimate stress.

Concerning changes of rhyme structures, the observed error patterns add further evidence to the assumption that metrical information of a phonological word

---

[3] In the metrical theory of German it remains unresolved so far whether a stray initial syllable creates a foot on its own or is left unparsed. The assumption that such syllables form monosyllabic feet poses a problem for the avoidance of stress clash, whereas an unparsed syllable violates the constraint that demands exhaustive parsing of syllables. Further research is necessary to validate the status of the two constraints involved.

influences the segmental make-up of a syllable. First of all, HT's phonological neologisms confirm that syllables bearing main stress are less error prone than syllables with secondary stress or weak syllables. This observation is in line with previous findings reported for example by Niemi et al. (1985) or Nickels and Howard (1999), who found aphasic omission errors mainly in unstressed syllables. Detailed analyses revealed that weak syllables were more prone to rhyme reduction, whereas syllables in head positions tended to become more complex. This finding is in line with suggestions concerning the relevance of rhyme structure for the phonetic prominence of a syllable, even for syllables that do not bear main stress (Alber, 1997, 1998; Féry, 1998; Giegerich, 1985).

It may be argued that in our study the metrical status of a syllable is just a confound with another factor, i.e., syllable frequency. According to this argument, less frequent syllables might have been replaced by syllables of higher frequency. Indeed, Aichert and Ziegler (2004b) found that the vulnerability of syllables in articulation crucially depended on syllable frequency in patients with apraxia of speech. With respect to impairments of phonological encoding in aphasia, Laganaro (2005) observed more errors in low-frequency syllables compared to high-frequency syllables. Stenneken, Hofmann, and Jacobs (2005) reported a preferred use of high-frequency compared to low-frequency syllables (see also Stenneken, Hofmann, & Jacobs, 2008 this issue). In both apraxia of speech and aphasia, effects of syllable frequency were interpreted as evidence for the existence of a syllabary involved in articulatory encoding during speech production. In order to investigate whether the observed changes in syllable structure reported in this paper are due to syllable frequency, we compared the frequency of each target syllable with the frequency of the corresponding paraphasic syllable (syllable frequencies calculated on the basis of the CELEX database—Baayen, Piepenbrock, & Gulikers, 1995—by Aichert, Marquardt, & Ziegler, unpublished). In fact, reduction errors, which mainly occurred in weak syllables, led to higher-frequent syllables (mean syllable frequency: target = 2332, response = 11076; Wilcoxon: $z = -4227, p < .001$). However, addition errors in syllables with secondary stress led to syllables that are numerically *less* frequent than the target (mean syllable frequency: target = 1405, response = 1113; Wilcoxon: $z = -.954, p > .34$). Thus, syllable frequency can be excluded as the only factor that influences the distribution of segment omissions, reductions, or insertions. Rather, the different patterns of segmental errors found in the three different syllable types speak in favour of a correlation between the prosodic status of a syllable and its segmental make-up.

Conclusion

To summarise, data from both reading and repetition indicate that the prosodic structure of German nouns is determined by segmental information, and therefore the encoding of segmental and metrical information cannot be completely independent in phonological encoding, as proposed by Levelt et al. (1999). On the one hand, the presence or absence of a coda consonant in final syllables designates either a final non-branching foot or a final trochee, surfacing as ultimate and antepenultimate stress or penultimate stress. On the other hand, regularisation errors have shown that words with penultimate stress optimally consist of an even number of syllables, whereas words with final or antepenultimate stress are preferably odd numbered. Thus, assumptions of metrical theory, e.g., leftward parsing of syllables into feet and the special status of unparsed syllables, have been supported (Alber, 1997, 1998). Finally, the degree of phonetic prominence of a syllable influences the probability of segments being omitted or inserted, speaking in favour of quantity-sensitive approaches of German word stress (Féry, 1998; Giegerich, 1985; Janßen, 2003a).

REFERENCES

Aichert, I., & Ziegler, W. (2004a). Segmental and metrical encoding in aphasia: Two case reports. *Aphasiology*, *18*, 1201–1211.

Aichert, I., & Ziegler, W. (2004b). Syllable frequency and syllable structure in apraxia of speech. *Brain and Language*, *88*, 148–159.

Aichert, I., Marquardt, C., & Ziegler, W. (unpublished). *German database for sublexical frequencies and structure*.

Alber, B. (1997). Quantity sensitivity as the result of constraint interaction. In G. E. Booij & J. v. d. Weijer (Eds.), *Phonology in progress – progress in phonology. HIL Phonology Paters III* (pp. 1–45). The Hague: Holland Academic Graphics.

Alber, B. (1998). Stress preservation in German loan words. In W. Kehrein & R. Wiese (Eds.), *Phonology and morphology of the Germanic languages* (pp. 113–141). Tübingen: Max Niemeyer Verlag.

Baayen, R. H., Piepenbrock, R., & Gulikers, L. (1995). *The CELEX Lexical Database, Release 2* [CD-ROM]. Linguistic Data Consortium, University of Pennsylvania, Philadelphia, PA.

Cappa, S., Nespor, M., Ielasi, W., & Miozzo, A. (1997). The representation of stress: Evidence from an aphasic patient. *Cognition*, *65*, 1–13.

De Bleser, R., Stadie, N., Tabatabaie, S., & Cholewa, J. (2004). *LeMo-Lexikon: Modell-orientierte Einzelfalldiagnostik bei Aphasie, Dyslexie und Dysgraphie*. München: Urban & Fischer.

Domahs, F., Bartha, L., Lochy, A., Benke, T., & Delazer, M. (2006). Number words are special: Evidence from a case of primary progressive aphasia. *Journal of Neurolinguistics*, *19*, 1–37.

Eisenberg, P. (1991). Syllabische Struktur und Wortakzent: Prinzipien der Prosodik deutscher Wörter. *Zeitschrift für Sprachwissenschaft*, *10*, 37–64.

Féry, C. (1998). German word stress in optimality theory. *Journal of Comparative Germanic Linguistics*, *2*, 101–142.

Gallante, E., Tralli, A., Zuffi, M., & Avanzi, S. (2000). Primary progressive aphasia: A patient with stress assignment impairment in reading aloud. *Neurological Science*, *21*, 39–48.

Gerken, L. A. (1996). Prosodic patterns in young children's language production. *Language*, *72*, 683–712.

Giegerich, H. J. (1985). *Metrical phonology and phonological structure*. Cambridge, UK: Cambridge University Press.

Hayes, B. (1995). *Metrical stress theory: Principles and case studies*. Chicago: University of Chicago Press.

Howard, D., & Smith, K. (2002). The effects of lexical stress in aphasic word production. *Aphasiology*, *16*, 198–237.

Huber, W., Poeck, K., Weniger, D., & Willmes, K. (1983). *Aachener Aphasie Test (AAT)*. Göttingen: Hogrefe.

Janßen, U. (2003a). *Untersuchungen zum Wortakzent im Deutschen und Niederländischen*. doctoral dissertation University of Duesseldorf, online dissertation available via URL: http://www.ub. uni-duesseldorf.de/home/etexte/diss/show?dissid=911).

Janßen, U. (2003b). Stress assignment in German patients with surface dyslexia. *Brain and Language*, *87*, 114–115.

Kager, R. (1989). *A metrical theory of stress and destressing in English and Dutch*. Dordrecht: Foris.

Kaltenbacher, E. (1994). Typologische Aspekte des Wortakzents: Zum Zusammenhang von Akzentposition und Silbengewicht im Arabischen und im Deutschen. *Zeitschrift für Sprachwissenschaft*, *13*, 20–55.

Kiparsky, P. (1979). Metrical structure assignment is cyclic. *Linguistic Inquiry*, *10*, 421–441.

Laganaro, M. (2005). Syllable frequency effect in speech production: Evidence from aphasia. *Journal of Neurolinguistics*, *18*, 221–235.

Laganaro, M., Vacheresse, F., & Frauenfelder, U. H. (2002). Selective impairment of lexical stress assignment in an Italian-speaking aphasic patient. *Brain and Language*, *81*, 601–609.

Langdon, D. W., & Warrington, E. K. (1995). *VESPAR – Verbal and Spatial Reasoning Test*. Hove, UK: Lawrence Erlbaum Associates Ltd.

Levelt, W. J. M. (1999). Models of word production. *Trends in Cognitive Sciences, 3*, 223–232.

Levelt, W. J. M., Roelofs, A., & Meyer, A. S. (1999). A theory of lexical access in speech production. *Behavioral and Brain Sciences, 22*, 1–75.

Liberman, M., & Prince, A. (1977). On stress and linguistic rhythm. *Linguistic Inquiry, 8*, 249–336.

Marshall, J. C., & Newcombe, F. G. (1973). Pattern of paralexia: A psycholinguistic approach. *Journal of Psycholinguistic Research, 2*, 175–199.

Mesulam, M. (2001). Primary progressive aphasia. *Annals of Neurology, 49*, 425–432.

Miceli, G., & Caramazza, A. (1993). The assignment of word stress in oral reading: Evidence form a case of acquired dyslexia. *Cognitive Neuropsychology, 10*, 273–296.

Nickels, L. A. (1997). Spoken word production and its breakdown in aphasia. Hove, UK: Psychology Press.

Nickels, L., & Howard, D. (1999). Effects of lexical stress on aphasic word production. *Clinical Linguistics and Phonetics, 13*, 269–294.

Niemi, J., Koivuselka-Sallinen, P., & Hanninen, R. (1985). Phoneme errors in Broca's aphasia: Three Finnish cases. *Brain and Language, 26*, 28–48.

Osterreith, P. A. (1944). Le test de copie d'une figure complexe. *Archives de Psychologie, 30*, 206–356.

Rey, A. (1941). L'examen psychologique dans le cas d'éncephalopathie traumatique. *Archives de Psychologie, 28*, 286–340.

Selkirk, E. O. (1982). The syllable. In H. van der Hulst & N. Smith (Eds.), *The structure of phonological representations (Part II)* (pp. 337–383). Dordrecht: Foris.

Stenneken, P., Hofmann, M., & Jacobs, A. M. (2005). Patterns of phoneme and syllable frequency in jargon aphasia. *Brain and Language, 95*, 221–222.

Stenneken, P., Hofmann, M., & Jacobs, A. M. (2008). Sublexical units in aphasic jargon and in the standard language. Comparative analyses of neologisms in connected speech. *Aphasiology, 22*, 1142–1156.

Wiese, R. (1996). *The phonology of German*. Oxford, UK: Oxford University Press.

APHASIOLOGY, 2008, 22 (11), 1176–1190

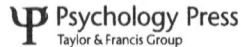

Syllabic processing in visual word recognition in Alzheimer patients, elderly people, and young adults

Manuel Carreiras

Universidad de La Laguna, Tenerife, Spain

Silvia Baquero

Universidad de La Laguna, Tenerife, Spain, and Universidad Nacional de Colombia, Colombia

Esperanza Rodríguez

Universidad Nacional de Colombia, Colombia

Background: Over the last decade Carreiras and colleages have assembled compelling empirical evidence that the syllable plays an important role in the visual recognition of polysyllabic words in Spanish. One of the clearest demonstrations of this is the *syllable frequency effect*: Words with high-frequency syllables are responded to more slowly than words with low-frequency syllables. Another key finding is the *syllable congruency effect* that has been obtained using the masked priming technique: Word recognition is facilitated by primes that correspond to the first syllable, relative to primes that contain one letter more or less than the first syllable.
Aims: The study aimed to investigate the syllable frequency effect and the syllable congruency effect in Alzheimer patients, elderly people, and young adults. The goal was to examine whether and to what extent syllabic processing is preserved or deteriorates with age and/or this disease. If structural components of language are to some extent preserved in Alzheimer's disease (AD) patients and in elderly people, they should show the syllable congruency effect. If AD patients and elderly people have a breakdown in the ability to inhibit partially activated information, the syllable frequency effect may well turn out to be different in these two groups as compared to the young adults.
Methods & Procedures: Two experiments, one investigating the syllable frequency effect and the other the syllable congruency effect, were carried out with Alzheimer patients, elderly people, and young adults. In Experiment 1 we used the same materials and procedure used by Carreiras and Perea (2002) in their Experiment 4. In Experiment 2 we created new materials manipulating syllable frequency (high and low) and word frequency (high and low). AD patients, elderly people, and young controls participated in the two experiments.
Outcomes & Results: The results showed syllable congruency effects, replicating previous findings. However, syllable frequency effects were different for the three groups. Predictably, young adults responded more slowly to words with high-frequency

---

Address correspondence to: Manuel Carreiras, Departamento de Psicología Cognitiva, Universidad de La Laguna, 38205-Tenerife, Spain. E-mail: mcarreir@ull.es

The research reported in this article has been partially supported by Grants SEJ2004-07680-C02-02/PSIC and SEJ2006-09238/PSIC from the Spanish Ministry of Education to MC and from the Spanish Agency of International cooperation (AECI) and Fundación Carolina to SB. We wish to thank Humberto Arboleda and Rodrigo Pardo of the *Grupo de Neurociencias de la Universidad Nacional de Colombia* for providing us with information about the patients' diagnosis profile and for kindly allowing us access to the patients.

---

http://www.psypress.com/aphasiology   DOI: 10.1080/02687030701820337

syllables than to words with low-frequency syllables. In contrast, Alzheimer patients and elderly people responded more slowly to words with low-frequency syllables than to words with high frequency syllables.

Conclusions: In the context of activation models that take into account a syllabic level of representation, the present results suggest that the syllabic layer is preserved but the inhibitory process of competition between lexical candidates is impaired in Alzheimer patients and in elderly people.

Keywords: visual word recognition; syllabic processing; Alzheimer; neurodegeneration; dementia.

Patients suffering from Alzheimer's disease (AD), a progressive neurodegenerative illness, exhibit impairments in memory, language processing, and other cognitive abilities. In fact, language dysfunction is recognised to be a central feature of the dementia in patients with a diagnosis of probable AD. However, while it is generally agreed that AD patients have a deficit in semantic processing (e.g., Bayles & Kaszniak, 1987; Cuetos, Martínez, Martínez, Izura, & Ellis, 2003; Hodges, Salmon, & Butters, 1992; Nebes, 1992; Nebes & Brady, 1991; Nestor, Scheltens, & Hodges, 2004), there are fewer data and there is much less consensus regarding the integrity of other language components such as syntax, morphology, phonology, and orthography (Bayles, Tomoeda, & Trosset, 1992; Cipolotti & Warrington, 1995; Cummings, Houlihan, & Hill, 1986; Friedman, Ferguson, Robinson, & Sunderland, 1992; Nebes, 1992; Patterson, Graham, & Hodges,1994a, 1994b). At the word level, persons with Alzheimer's disease (AD) demonstrate a severe lexical impairment that affects conceptual knowledge. Typically, patients manifest anomia (word-finding difficulty) and impairment in verbal fluency early in the course of the disease, suggesting that AD patients' linguistic impairment is a result of either damage to semantic knowledge or difficulty accessing the information stored there (for a review, see Caramelli, Mansur, & Nitrini, 1998). Many studies have documented impairments of word meaning in AD. For instance, persons with AD are often impaired in naming (e.g., Nicholas, Obler, Au, & Albert, 1996), and in word comprehension (e.g., Hodges et al., 1992). In addition, evidence for word-priming abnormalities has also been reported in this population (e.g., Bell, Chenery, & Ingram, 2001; Chertkow et al., 1994; Chertkow, Bub, & Seidenberg, 1989; Giffard et al., 2001; Margolin, Pate, & Friedrich, 1996). However, research into aspects of word structure has been scarce.

According to the results obtained in studies of semantic dementia, deterioration in conceptual knowledge can have an impact on lower-level orthographic and phonological processes. For example, it has been demonstrated that degraded semantics can affect the integrity of phonological word forms in the context of a verbal immediate serial recall task in semantic dementia (Jefferies, Patterson, Jones, Bateman, & Lambon Ralph, 2004; Knott, Patterson, & Hodges, 1997; Patterson, et al., 1994b). The negative impact of degraded semantic memory on phonological (and possibly orthographic) processing has also been demonstrated in word reading. Patients with semantic dementia commonly exhibit the acquired reading disorder known as surface dyslexia, in which they are prone to error in oral reading of words with atypical spelling–sound correspondences. All the patients with semantic dementia analysed by Woollams, Lambon Ralph, Hodges, and Patterson (2005) showed a surface dyslexic pattern of reading. However, it remains to be seen whether sublexical (orthographic-phonological) structural features such as syllables are deteriorated in AD patients during the early to middle course of the illness in a language with transparent orthography, such as Spanish, which has been repeatedly shown to be processed syllabically during reading of complex words in young adults (e.g., Carreiras, Alvarez, & de Vega, 1993; Carreiras & Perea, 2002; Perea & Carreiras, 1998). This is the goal of the present paper.

One of the key findings for the existence of syllabic processing in visual word recognition in Spanish is the syllable frequency effect—i.e., words composed of high-frequency syllables are responded to more slowly than words composed of low-frequency syllables in lexical decision (Carreiras et al., 1993; see also Alvarez, Carreiras, & Taft, 2001; Barber, Vergara, & Carreiras, 2004; Perea & Carreiras, 1998). The processing delay for words with high syllable frequency is interpreted to reflect interference caused by other word representations sharing the same syllable in the same position. This effect has also been replicated in other languages (German: Conrad & Jacobs, 2004; French: Mathey & Zagar, 2002). Interestingly, other potential explanatory factors of the syllable frequency effect have already been discarded: neither bigram frequency (Carreiras et al., 1993), orthographic neighbourhood density/frequency (Alvarez et al., 2001; Perea & Carreiras, 1998), nor morpheme frequency (Alvarez et al., 2001) can account for the previous findings. Converging evidence for the use of the first syllable as a sublexical unit has also been obtained with masked primes that share their initial syllable with the target word (Alvarez, Carreiras, & Perea, 2004; Carreiras & Perea, 2002; Carreiras, Ferrand, Grainger, & Perea, 2005a) or by presenting words in two colours so that the boundaries between the two colours and the boundaries between the first and the second syllable are either congruent or incongruent (Carreiras, Vergara, & Barber, 2005b). For instance, Carreiras and Perea (2002, Experiment 3) used monosyllabic (*ZINC*) and disyllabic words (*RA.NA*) as targets (the dots represent syllable boundaries.). The results showed a significant priming effect for disyllabic words (*ra.jo–RA.NA* relative to *cu.fo–RA.NA*). In contrast, monosyllabic words were not affected by related primes that shared the first two letters with the target (*ziel–ZINC* vs *flur–ZINC*). Likewise, in their Experiment 4 (see also Alvarez et al., 2004) Carreiras and Perea (2002) found a significant advantage for disyllabic prime–target pairs that shared the first syllable (e.g., pa****–<u>PA.SIVO</u>, pas***–<u>PAS.TOR</u>) relative to disyllabic pairs that did not share the first syllable (pas***–<u>PA.SIVO</u>, pa****–<u>PAS.TOR</u>). Further, in a recent paper with French stimuli, Carreiras et al. (2005a) found a significant masked priming effect for the phonological first syllable (*fo.mie–FAU.CON* vs *pe.mie–FAU.CON*) but not for the phonological second syllable (*re.tôt–GA.TEAU* vs *re.din–GA.TEAU*). Taken together, these masked priming experiments reinforce the view that the first syllable is the critical unit for syllabic effects to occur, at least in Romance languages. Furthermore, these findings provide additional evidence that syllables are relevant phonological input representations in visual word recognition.

While the syllable congruency effect may tap into earlier stages of word recognition, namely syllabification, the syllable frequency effect seems to be the end result of a late lexical inhibitory process. The effects of syllable frequency in the lexical decision task, indicating a processing delay for words with high-frequency syllables as compared to words with low-frequency syllables, has been interpreted to reflect interference caused by other word representations sharing the same syllable in the same position. It is assumed that after a syllabic segmentation of the input, the first syllable activates the representations of words sharing this syllable in identical position. High-frequency syllables are assumed to fire more lexical candidates than low-frequency syllables because a high-frequency syllable is shared by more words. This early firing of lexical candidates is followed by a competition process among the lexical candidates to suppress the activation of all candidates except the word that is recognised. Electrophysiological correlates of these two processes—early facilitation and late inhibition—manipulating syllable frequency have been obtained (Barber et al., 2004). It is important to note that there are two possible ways to compute syllable frequency: type and token. Most of the experiments that have been performed to date have manipulated syllable token frequency. Interestingly, Conrad, Carreiras, and Jacobs (2008) contrasted syllable token and type frequency and found a clear inhibitory effect of syllable frequency when selected according to token frequency. In the present experiment we manipulated syllable token frequency.

An impairment of inhibitory capacity has been observed in AD patients and elderly people above 65–70 years in different tasks (Amieva et al., 2002; Balota & Duchek, 1991; Faust, Balota, Duchek, Gernsbacher, & Smith, 1997; Hasher & Zacks, 1988; Spieler, Balota, & Faust, 1996; Sullivan, Faust, & Balota, 1995). In particular, Hasher and Zacks (1988) have suggested that healthy aged individuals have a breakdown in the ability to inhibit partially activated information, while Balota and colleages (e.g., Balota & Duchek, 1991; Balota & Ferraro, 1993; Sullivan et al., 1995) have argued that a similar framework may be useful in accounting for some of the cognitive deficits that are observed in individuals with AD. Therefore, if elderly people and AD patients show a breakdown in the ability to inhibit partially activated information, they should not show the inhibitory effects of syllable frequency. Instead, it is more likely that they show facilitatory effects of syllable frequency, which would reflect the earlier stages of activation of lexical candidates.

To investigate whether and to what extent syllabic processing is preserved or deteriorated in patients with AD, we carried out two experiments, one investigating the syllable congruency effect and the other the syllable frequency effect. In Experiment 1 we used the same materials and procedure used by Carreiras and Perea (2002) in their Experiment 4 with AD patients in early stages of the illness and a control group of elderly persons of similar age and level of education. If the structural components of language are to some extent preserved in AD patients and in elderly people, they should show the syllable congruency effect. In Experiment 2 we created new materials, manipulating syllable frequency (high and low) and word frequency (high and low) to investigate the syllable frequency effect in three groups: AD patients, elderly people, and young controls. If AD patients and elderly people have a breakdown in the ability to inhibit partially activated information, the syllable frequency effect may well turn out to be different in these two groups as compared to the young adults.

EXPERIMENT 1: SYLLABIC STRUCTURE

Method

Participants. We investigated a total of 16 seniors with an average age of 72.1 years (range: 53–87) and 16 patients with an average age of 72.6 years (range: 53–87) with probable Alzheimer disease. All were native speakers of Spanish. All participants had completed at least the sixth grade of schooling and had no history of learning disabilities or prior psychiatric illness. The AD patients and elderly controls did not differ in mean years of education or in age. The patients met NINCDS-ADRDA (National Institute of Neurological and Communicative Disorders and Stroke (NINCDS) and Alzheimer Disease and Related Disorders Association (ADRDA) research diagnostic criteria for probable AD (McKhann et al., 1984). All had undergone medical, neurological, and neurodiagnostic evaluations to ensure that the dementia symptoms could not be attributed to any other cause. The battery of neuropsychological evaluation included tests of verbal fluency, memory, picture naming, picture copy, intelligence, and executive function. Patients were evaluated by the "Grupo de Neurociencias" from the Universidad Nacional de Colombia. Dementia severity ranged from mild to moderately impaired. The mean score on the Mini-Mental State Examination (MMSE) (Folstein, Folstein, & McHugh, 1975) was 21.1 (range 18–24), and the mean score on the Global Deterioration Scale (GDS) (Reisberg et al., 1982) was 3.4 (range 3–4). Elderly controls were interviewed to ascertain that they had no neurological or major medical illness. The mean score on the MMSE was 28.8 (range 26–30) and on the GDS Scale it was 1.4 (range 1–2) in the elderly controls.

Materials. The materials were the same as those used in Experiment 4 of Carreiras and Perea (2002). A total of 80 six-letter Spanish words were selected from the Spanish word pool. According to the LEXESP database (Sebastián-Gallés, Martí, Carreiras, & Cuetos, 2000) 40 words had a CV.CV.CV structure (mean frequency: 18.6 per million words, range: 2–132) and 40 had a CVC.CVC structure (mean frequency: 16.4 per million words, range: 1–81). In addition, the number of neighbours in both conditions was similar according the B-Pal database (Davis & Perea, 2005): for CV.CV.CV words, 2.6 neighbours (range 0–9), and for CVC.CVC words, 1.3 neighbours (range 0–4). For each target word (or nonword), two types of prime were selected: (1) primes that corresponded to the first syllable (e.g., pa****_ PA.SIVO, pas***–PAS.TOR); (2) primes that did not correspond to the first syllable (pas***–PA.SIVO, pa****–PAS.TOR). Prime–target pairs were counterbalanced in two lists, so that no participant saw any target more than once, but each participant received the four experimental conditions (20 pairs per condition). In addition, 80 nonwords were created for the purposes of the lexical decision task. All of them were orthographically legal in Spanish. On half of the trials the primes corresponded to the first syllable, and on the other half the primes did not correspond to the first syllable (in an analogous way to word targets). Each participant was given a total of 160 experimental trials.

Design. Stimulus onset asynchrony, henceforth SOA (116 vs 166 ms) was varied between participants following the original experiment of Carreiras and Perea (2002). Eight patients and eight controls participated at the 116-ms SOA and the other eight patients and eight controls participated at the 166-ms SOA, whereas type of prime (CV vs CVC) and type of target (CV vs CVC structure) was varied within participants.

Procedure. Participants were tested individually in a quiet room. Presentation of the stimuli and recording of reaction times were controlled on a personal computer by a program in EXPE6 (Pallier, Dupoux, & Jeannin, 1997). On each trial, a forward mask consisting of six hash marks (######) was presented for 500 ms. This was immediately followed by presentation of the prime for 116 or 166 ms, followed immediately by presentation of the target item (in uppercase letters). The target remained on the screen until the participant responded. The computer recorded the lexical decision times, measured from target onset until the participant's response. Participants were instructed to press one of two buttons on the keyboard ("M" for yes and "Z" for no) to indicate as rapidly and as accurately as possible whether the uppercase letter string was a legitimate Spanish word or not. After the participant's response, the target disappeared from the screen. After an inter-trial interval of 1500 ms, the next trial was presented. Stimulus presentation was randomised, with a different order for each participant. Each participant received a total of 48 practice trials prior to the 160 experimental trials.

Results and discussion

Incorrect responses (6.3% for patients and 4.5% for controls) were excluded from the latency analysis. In addition, reaction times more than 2.0 standard deviations above or below the mean for that participant in all conditions were also excluded. The percentage of trials that were removed was similar in the CV and the CVC priming conditions. For patients, for CVC target words, these percentages were 11.2% and 11.6% for the CV and the CVC primes, respectively; whereas for CV target words these percentages were 9.2% and 9.4% for the CV and the CVC primes, respectively. For controls, for CVC target words, these percentages were 9.1% and 9.4% for the CV and the CVC primes, respectively; whereas for CV target words these percentages were 7.8% and 8.4% for the CV and the CVC primes, respectively.

For each group of participants (patients and elderly), participant and item ANOVAs based on the participant (F1) and item (F2) response latencies and percentage of errors were conducted based on a 2 (SOA: 116, 166) $\times$ 2 (Type of prime: CV, CVC) $\times$ 2 (Type of target: CV.CV.CV, CVC.CVC) design. The mean lexical decision time and the error rate on the stimulus words in each experimental condition are shown in Table 1.

Alzheimer patients. The ANOVA on the latency data showed a significant main effect of SOA, $F1(1, 15) = 1.4, p > 10; F2(1, 76) = 61.1, p < .001$, so that target words at the SOA of 116 were slower (1768) than at the SOA of 166 ms (1431).

The ANOVAs on the latency data showed a significant interaction between Type of target and Type of prime, $F1(1, 15) = 3.48, p < .10 F2(1, 76) = 75.5, p < .001$: CVC.CVC words were responded to faster when preceded by CVC primes than when preceded by CV primes, $F1(1, 15) = 3.1, p < .10; F2(1, 76) = 75.2, p < .001$. In contrast, CV.CV.CV words were responded to faster when preceded by CV primes than when preceded by CVC primes, $F1(1, 15) = 3.7, p < .10; F2(1, 76) = 81.3, p < .001$.

The ANOVA on the error data only showed a significant interaction between Type of target and Type of prime, $F1(1, 15) = 7.4, p < .05; F2(1, 76) = 16.8, p < .001$: CVC.CVC words were responded to with a lower percentage of errors when preceded by CVC primes than when preceded by CV primes, $F1(1, 15) = 3.5, p < .10; F2(1, 76) = 6.5, p < .05$. In contrast, CV.CV.CV words were responded to with a lower percentage of errors when preceded by CV primes than when preceded by CVC primes, $F1(1, 15) = 10.7, p < .01; F2(1, 76) = 10.7, p < .001$. The other main effects and interactions were not significant (all $ps > .10$).

TABLE 1
Experiment 1

	Type of prime		
	CV	CVC	CVC-CV
	Alzheimer patients		
SOA = 116 ms			
CV structure	1607 (3.2)	2260 (9.1)	653 (5.9)
CVC structure	2225 (11.1)	1590 (6.3)	−635(−4.8)
SOA = 166 ms			
CV structure	1192 (3.5)	1770 (9.8)	578 (6.3)
CVC structure	1725 (7.6)	1147 (4.1)	−578 (−3.5)
	Elderly controls		
SOA = 116 ms			
CV structure	925 (2.0)	1055 (5.1)	103(3.1)
CVC structure	1059 (5.2)	889 (4.3)	−170(−0.9)
SOA = 166 ms			
CV structure	989 (2.8)	1377 (4.0)	388 (1.2)
CVC structure	1311 (4.6)	991 (5.3)	−320 (−0.7)

Mean lexical decision times (in ms) and percentage of errors (in parentheses) on target words in Experiment 1.

Elderly people. The ANOVAs on the latency data showed the main effect of SOA, $F1(1, 14) = 6.0, p < .05; F2(1, 76) = 34.7, p < .001$, so that target words were faster at SOA 116 (980) than at 166 (1167).

More importantly, there was a significant interaction between Type of target and Type of prime, $F1(1, 14) = 9.7, p < .01; F2(1, 76) = 35. 9, p < .001$: CVC.CVC words were responded to faster when preceded by CVC primes than when preceded by CV primes, $F1(1, 14) = 12.4, p < .01; F2(1, 76) = 14.8, p < .001$. In contrast, CV.CV.CV words were responded to faster when preceded by CV primes than when preceded by CVC primes, $F1(1, 14) = 7.2, p < .05; F2(1, 76) = 21.6, p < .001$. The other main effects and interactions were not significant (all $ps > .10$).

The ANOVA on the error data yielded no significant main effects or interactions (all $ps > .10$).

Since the pattern of data in terms of syllable congruency is similar for the two groups of participants, even though some effects are not significant in the analysis by participants in the case of the patients, we performed an analysis including group as a new variable to increase statistical power in the analysis by participants. This showed a clear effect of syllable congruency in the interaction prime × target both in reaction times, $F1(1, 28) = 6.1, p < .05; F2(1, 76) = 73.5, p < .001$, and in error rates, $F1(1, 28) = 8.2, p < .01; F2(1, 76) = 15.7, p < .001$.

Discussion

The results of this experiment are straightforward. There was a clear syllable congruency effect: CV.CV.CV targets preceded by CV primes were responded to faster than those preceded by CVC primes, whereas CVC.CVC targets preceded by

CVC primes were responded to faster than those preceded by CV primes. This finding extends the data obtained by Carreiras and Perea (2002) and reveals that this early process is preserved in elderly controls and in the AD patients. Of course, reading times are much longer in these two groups than those observed with undergraduates in Carreiras and Perea (2002). However, the important result is that the same pattern of syllabic congruency appears in the three groups of participants. Importantly, this reinforces the view that sublexical input phonology is structured syllabically, at least for languages with clear syllable boundaries (see Alvarez et al., 2001; Carreiras et al., 1993; Ferrand, Segui, & Grainger, 1996; Perea & Carreiras, 1998). Nonetheless, even though AD patients and elderly people seem to be able to segment the input words in syllables, and activate lexical candidates according to this segmentation, they can experience problems later, at the stage at which inhibitory processes need to be working to select the right lexical candidate. This is the goal of Experiment 2, in which we manipulated the syllable frequency.

EXPERIMENT 2: SYLLABLE FREQUENCY

Method

Participants. Participants were 20 undergraduate students from the National University of Colombia with an average age of 21.7 years (range 19–25), 20 seniors with an average age of 71.6 years (range 65–83), and 20 patients with probable Alzheimer Disease with an average age of 72.7 years (range 53 to 85). All were native speakers of Spanish. All participants had completed at least the sixth grade of schooling and had no history of learning disabilities or prior psychiatric illness. The patients met NINCDS-ADRDA research diagnostic criteria for probable AD (McKhann et al., 1984). All had undergone medical, neurological, and neurodiagnostic evaluations to ensure that the dementia symptoms could not be attributed to any other cause. The battery of neuropsychological evaluation included tests of verbal fluency, memory, picture naming, picture copy, intelligence, and executive function. Patients were evaluated by the "Grupo de Neurociencias" from the Universidad Nacional de Colombia. Dementia severity ranged from mild to moderate. For AD patients the mean score on the MMSE was 20.6 (range 19–24) and the mean score on the GDS Scale was 3.8 (range 3–4). Elderly controls were interviewed to ascertain that they had no neurological or major medical illness. The AD and elderly control groups did not differ in mean years of education or in age. The mean score on the MMSE was 27.8 (range 25–30) and the mean score on the GDS Scale was 1.8 (range 1–2).

Materials. The stimuli were 48 disyllabic Spanish words, all of them of four or five letters. The words had been selected by combining two variables (syllable frequency of the first syllable: low vs high; word frequency: low vs high) in a 2 × 2 within-participants but between-items design. We selected syllables according to their token positional frequency in the dictionary of frequency of syllables in Spanish (Sebastián-Gallés et al., 2000). We considered words to be of high frequency when they had a minimum frequency of occurrence of 32 per million (range 32–676), and to be of low frequency when they had a maximum frequency of occurrence of 11 per million (range 2–11). We considered syllables to be of high frequency when they had a minimum token frequency of occurrence in first position of 3235 (range 3235–42914) per million in the Spanish database, and to be of low frequency when they had a maximum token frequency of occurrence in first position of 1582 (range 155–1582). The positional frequency of each syllable refers to the number of times that the syllable (weighted by lexical frequency) appeared in that word position (first, second, final, etc.). To control for the bigram trough (see Rapp, 1992), the bigram that crossed the two syllables (e.g., *ob* in the word *lo.bo*) had a higher or equal positional (token) bigram frequency than the average of the neighbouring bigrams (i.e., the average of the positional token bigram frequencies of *lo* and *bo*). Syllabic structure was matched across the four conditions and words were also matched across conditions for the number of letters (average of 5; range 4–6) and for the number of orthographic neighbours (average of 7; range 0–25). In addition, for the purpose of the lexical decision task, we created a set of 48 pseudowords of similar length, bigram trough ratio, and number of neighbours as those of the words.

Procedure. Participants were tested individually in a quiet room. Presentation of the stimuli and recording of response times were controlled in a PC compatible computer by a program in EXPE6. Participants were told that words and nonwords would be displayed on the monitor in front of them, and that they should press one of two buttons ("M" for yes and "Z" for no) to indicate whether each stimulus was a word or a nonword, responding as rapidly as possible while maintaining a reasonable level of accuracy. On each trial, an asterisk was presented for 500 ms, which was immediately followed by presentation of the stimuli (word or nonword). Stimuli were presented in lower case and remained visible until the participant responded. The computer recorded the lexical decision times, measured from target onset until the participant's response. When the participant responded, the target disappeared from the screen. After an inter-trial interval of 1000 ms, the next trial was presented. Stimulus presentation was randomised, with a different order for each participant. Each participant received a total of 30 practice trials prior to the 96 experimental trials.

Results and discussion

Incorrect responses (6.2% for patients, 4.9% for elderly people, 3.1% for young participants) were excluded from the latency analysis. In addition, in order to avoid the influence of outliers, all reaction times more than 2.0 standard deviations above or below the mean for that participant in all conditions were also excluded. The percentage of trials that were removed was similar in all conditions. For words, these percentages were 8.9%, 8.2 %, and 4.1% for AD patients, elderly people, and young participants respectively.

Participant and item ANOVAs based on the participant and item response latencies and percentage of errors were conducted based on a 2 (word frequency: high and low) × 2 (Syllable frequency: high and low) design for each group separately. The mean lexical decision times and the percentage of errors on the words in each experimental condition for each group are displayed in Table 2.

Alzheimer patients. The ANOVA on the latency data showed that only the main effect of lexical frequency was significant in the items analysis, $F1(1, 17) < 1$; $F2 (1, 45) = 10.3, p < .01$. The main effect of syllable frequency and the interaction were not

TABLE 2
Experiment 2

	Alzheimer patients		Elderly controls		Young controls	
	HFS	LFS	HFS	LFS	HFS	LFS
HFW	1518 (3.6)	1565 (5.0)	1409 (2.6)	1475 (3.0)	641 (1.6)	623 (0.3)
LFW	1537 (7.8)	1614 (6.8)	1524 (5.6)	1621(4.8)	713 (3.4)	655 (0.8)

Mean lexical decision times (in ms) and percentage of errors (in parentheses) on words in Experiment 2. HFW = High-frequency words. LFW = Low-frequency words. HFS = High-frequency syllables. LFS = Low-frequency syllables.

significant (all $ps > .10$). The ANOVA on error rates did not show any significant effects; only lexical frequency was marginally significant in the analysis by subjects, $F1(1, 17) = 3.9$, $p < .10$; $F2 < 1$.

Elderly people. The ANOVA on the latency data showed that, on average, participants classified high-frequency words faster than low-frequency words, $F1(1, 17) = 29.1$, $p < .001$; $F2(1, 45) = 7.1$, $p < .05$. In addition, participants classified words with high-frequency syllables faster than words with low-frequency syllables, $F1(1, 17) = 4.7$, $p < .05$; $F2(1, 45) = 2.9$, $p < .10$. The interaction between word and syllable frequency was not significant ($p > .10$). The ANOVA on error rates did not show any significant effects.

Young people. The ANOVA on the latency data showed that, on average, participants classified high-frequency words faster than low-frequency words, $F1(1, 17) = 32.8$, $p < .001$; $F2(1, 45) = 4.1$, $p < .05$. In addition, participants classified words with high-frequency syllables slower than words with low-frequency syllables, $F1(1, 17) = 10.8$, $p < .05$; $F2(1, 45) = 6.3$, $p < .05$. The interaction between the two variables was not significant, $F1(1, 17) = 1.5$, $F2 < 1$.

The ANOVA on the error rates showed that participants classified high-frequency words more accurately than low-frequency words, $F1(1, 17) = 37.8$, $p < .001$; $F2(1, 45) = 5.9$, $p < .05$. In addition, participants classified words with high-frequency syllables less accurately than words with low-frequency syllables, $F1(1, 17) = 28.0$, $p < .05$; $F2(1, 45) = 11.5$, $p < .001$. In addition, the interaction between word and syllable frequency was significant, $F1(1, 17) = 25.0$, $p < .001$; $F2 < 1$, indicating that the effects of syllable frequency were larger for low-frequency words, $F1(1, 18) = 39.1$, $p < .001$, than for high-frequency words, $F1(1, 17) = 13.4$, $p < .001$, although in both cases syllable frequency remains significant .

Clearly, the pattern of data of the young participants differs from that of the AD patients and the elderly people. In addition, the pattern of data of the elderly people and the AD patients is quite similar. However, we were unable to observe significant differences in the group of AD patients because of the high variability in this group and the scarce number of participants. Therefore, to increase our statistical power we performed a new analysis with the two groups (AD patients and elderly people). The ANOVA showed a main effect of lexical frequency: participants classified high-frequency words faster than low-frequency words, $F1(1, 35) = 7.4$, $p \leqslant .01$; $F2(1, 45) = 14.5$, $p < .001$. In addition, participants classified words with high-frequency syllables faster than the words with low-frequency syllables, $F1(1, 35) = 5.7$, $p < .05$;

$F2(1, 45) = 1.6, p > .10$. Furthermore, the main effect of group was significant in the item analysis, $F1(1, 35) < 1$; $F2(1, 45) = 27.9, p < .001$. None of the interactions was significant. In addition, the ANOVA on error rates showed that participants classified high-frequency words more accurately than low-frequency words, $F1(1, 35) = 7.4, p \leqslant .01$; $F2(1, 45) = 3.3, p < .10$. None of the other effects was significant.

The outcome of the present experiment showed a clear inhibitory effect of syllable frequency for the young controls, whereas no inhibition at all was found for the other two groups (elderly people and AD patients)—indeed, instead there was a facilitatory pattern. Since facilitation instead of inhibition has been obtained in the elderly people and the AD patients, this result provides evidence in favour of the breakdown of inhibitory abilities in these two populations. In fact, this behavioural pattern of data could result from effects originating in earlier processes of activation that have been observed with electrophysiological measures in young populations. This activation stage could last longer in the AD patients and the elderly people, due to the lack of sufficient inhibitory mechanisms.

GENERAL DISCUSSION

The main findings of the present experiments can be summarised as follows: (i) Syllable congruency effects were obtained in AD patients and in elderly people; (ii) inhibitory syllable frequency effects were obtained in young controls, but facilitatory effects were obtained in AD patients and in elderly people; (iii) The usual word frequency effect was obtained in the three groups of participants, although the effects were not significant in the by-subjects analysis in the group of AD patients; (iv) as expected, reaction times were longer in the AD patients and elderly people than in the young controls.

The longer reaction times of the elderly people and AD patients are consistent with those of many other experiments showing that healthy older adults are more error prone and show slower processing (e.g., Balota & Ferraro, 1996; Taylor & Burke; 2002). Regarding the lexical frequency effects, there has been some recent controversy concerning word frequency effects in young and older adults (see Balota & Ferraro, 1996). For instance Allen, Madden, Weber, and Groth (1993) have claimed that there is no change in the word frequency effect between young individuals and healthy, aged individuals. However, Balota and Ferraro (1993) provided evidence of an increasing word frequency effect in AD patients as compared to elderly healthy individuals, and Balota and Ferraro (1996) found that the word frequency effect in lexical decision performance was larger in the healthy older adults than in the healthy younger adults under conditions in which verbal WAIS-R performance was equated. In the present experiment, there is a larger word frequency effect in the elderly healthy individuals as compared to the young controls. However, the AD patients showed a reduced word frequency effect, ever smaller than the young controls. Since we have not controlled for vocabulary scores between the three groups of participants, it could be claimed that vocabulary size could be responsible for the observed differences. Nonetheless, even though vocabulary size could be different between the young controls and the other two groups, the AD patients and elderly people were equivalent in years of schooling, which could be related to some extent to vocabulary size, and they have shown a very different word frequency size. Thus, our data are consistent with the proposal that word frequency effects increase with age, but they do not replicate other studies (e.g., Balota &

Ferraro, 1993) that have also observed an increase of the word frequency effect with AD patients.

The observed syllable congruency effects are consistent with the previous data obtained by Carreiras and Perea (2002) with young undergraduates, suggesting that syllabic segmentation, a structural level of language, is preserved in these two groups. These data are also consistent with the idea that some structural components of language remain preserved in elderly people and in moderate stages of Alzheimer's disease.

Regarding the syllable frequency effects, a particularly interesting finding was that of equivalent facilitatory effects in AD patients and elderly people, but different from the young controls, who showed the typical inhibitory effect. These results suggest that the lexically interrelated alternative lexical items that are activated during the initial stage of lexical access are not being suppressed. The finding of a facilitatory effect of syllable frequency adds positive support to the claims of a general inhibitory breakdown with age (e.g., Hasher, Zacks, & Rahhal, 1999; Zacks & Hasher, 1994). Only young adults were able to exert inhibitory control over inappropriate information—lexical competitors that shared the first syllable.

The hypothesis of a general inhibitory control deficit for either healthy ageing or AD patients has been supported by an important set of previous data using different tasks. For example, studies of Stroop colour naming (Spieler et al., 1996), phonological processing (e.g., Balota & Ferraro, 1993, 1996), sentence comprehension and homograph priming (e.g., Balota & Duchek, 1991; Faust et al., 1997), and recovery from garden path sentences (Hartman & Hasher, 1991; May, Zacks, Hasher, & Multhaup, 1999), among others, have demonstrated age-related decrements in inhibitory control. Our results are also consistent with more general claims that AD-related breakdowns in inhibitory cognitive mechanisms are associated with executive attention (e.g., Balota & Faust, 2001). Balota and Faust suggested that declines in inhibition associated with AD seem to be related with the attentional control mechanisms responsible for, among other things, selection of a relevant subset of information under conditions in which irrelevant information is active, and selection of relevant behavioural responses in situations with several active alternatives. In any case, our data show that while efficient processing includes both the activation of relevant representations and the inhibition of partially relevant but incorrect representations or selection through attentional control mechanisms, elderly people and AD patients seem to be inefficient in the later selection stage.

In sum, we report evidence showing a preservation of structural sublexical information and a significant difference in the suppression of lexical information. Therefore, our data are consistent with an age-related breakdown in inhibitory mechanisms that may be more serious in AD.

REFERENCES

Allen, P. A., Madden, D. J., Weber, T. A., & Groth, K. E. (1993). Influence of age and processing stage on visual word recognition. *Psychology and Aging, 8,* 274–282.

Alvarez, C. J., Carreiras, M., & Perea, M. (2004). Are syllables phonological units in visual word recognition? *Language and Cognitive Processes, 9,* 427–452.

Alvarez, C. J., Carreiras, M., & Taft, M. (2001). Syllables and morphemes: Contrasting frequency effects in Spanish. *Journal of Experimental Psychology. Learning, Memory, and Cognition, 27,* 545–555.

Amieva, H. L. N., Lafont, S., Auriacombe, S., Le Carret, N., Dartigues, J., & Orgogozo, J. M. et al. (2002). Inhibitory breakdown and dementia of the Alzheimer type: A general phenomenon? *Journal of Clinical & Experimental Neuropsychology, 24,* 503.

Balota, D. A., & Duchek, J. M. (1991). Semantic priming effects, lexical repetition effects, and contextual disambiguation effects in healthy aged individuals and individuals with senile dementia of the Alzheimer type. *Brain and Language, 40,* 181–201.

Balota, D. A., & Faust, M. (2001). Attention in dementia of the Alzheimer type. In F. Boller & S. Cappa (Eds.), *Handbook of neuropsychology.* (2nd ed., Vol. 6, pp. 51–80). Amsterdam: Elsevier Science.

Balota, D. A., & Ferraro, F. R. (1993). A dissociation of frequency and regularity effects in pronunciation performance across young adults, older adults, and individuals with senile dementia of the Alzheimer type. *Journal of Memory and Language, 32,* 573–592.

Balota, D. A., & Ferraro, F. R. (1996). Lexical, sublexical, and implicit memory processes in healthy young, healthy older adults, and in individuals with dementia of the Alzheimer's type. *Neuropsychology, 10,* 82–95.

Barber, H., Vergara, M., & Carreiras, M. (2004). Syllable-frequency effects in visual word recognition: Evidence from ERPs. *Neuroreport, 15,* 545–548.

Bayles, K. A., & Kaszniak, A. W. (1987). *Communication and cognition in normal aging and dementia.* Boston, MA: Little, Brown & Co.

Bayles, K. A., Tomoeda, C. K., & Trosset, M. W. (1992). Relation of linguistic communication abilities of Alzheimer's patients to stage of disease. *Brain and Language, 42,* 454–472.

Bell, E. E., Chenery, H. J., & Ingram, J. C. L. (2001). Semantic priming in Alzheimer's dementia: Evidence for dissociation of automatic and attentional processes. *Brain and Language, 76,* 130–144.

Caramelli, P., Mansur, L. L., & Nitrini, R. (1998). Language and communication disorders in dementia of the Alzheimer's type. In B. Stemmer & H. Whitaker (Eds.), *Handbook of neurolinguistics* (pp. 463–473). San Diego, CA: Academic Press.

Carreiras, M., Alvarez, C. J., & de Vega, M. (1993). Syllable frequency and visual word recognition in Spanish. *Journal of Memory and Language, 32,* 766–780.

Carreiras, M., & Perea, M. (2002). Masked priming effects with syllabic neighbours in a lexical decision task. *Journal of Experimental Psychology. Human Perception and Performance, 28,* 1228–1242.

Carreiras, M., Ferrand, L., Grainger, J., & Perea, M. (2005a). Sequential effects of phonological priming in visual word recognition. *Psychological Science, 16,* 585–589.

Carreiras, M., Vergara, M., & Barber, H. (2005b). Early ERP effects of syllabic processing during visual word recognition. *Journal of Cognitive Neuroscience, 18,* 1803–1817.

Chertkow, H., Bub, D., Bergman, H., Bruemmer, A., Merling, A., & Rothfleisch, J. (1994). Increased semantic priming in patients with dementia of the Alzheimer's type. *Journal of Clinical Experimental Neuropsychology, 16,* 608–622.

Chertkow, H., Bub, D., & Seidenberg, M. (1989). Priming and semantic memory loss in Alzheimer's disease. *Brain and Language, 36,* 420.

Cipolotti, L., & Warrington, E. K. (1995). Towards a unitary account of access dysphasia: A single case study. *Memory, 3,* 309–332.

Conrad, M., Carreiras, M., & Jacobs, A. (2008). Contrasting effects of token and type syllable frequency in lexical decision. *Language and Cognitive Processes, 23,* 1–31.

Conrad, M., & Jacobs, A. M. (2004). Replicating syllable frequency effects in Spanish in German: One more challenge to computational models of visual word recognition. *Language & Cognitive Processes, 19,* 369–390.

Cuetos, F., Martinez, T., Martinez, C., Izura, C., & Ellis, A. W. (2003). Lexical processing in Spanish patients with probable Alzheimer's disease. *Brain Research. Cognitive Brain Research, 17,* 549–561.

Cummings, J. L., Houlihan, J. P., & Hill, M. A. (1986). The pattern of reading deterioration in dementia of the Alzheimer type: Observations and implications. *Brain and Language, 29,* 315–323.

Davis, C. J., & Perea, M. (2005). BuscaPalabras: A program for deriving orthographic and phonological neighbourhood statistics and other psycholinguistic indices in Spanish. *Behavior Research Methods, 37,* 665–671.

Faust, M. E., Balota, D. A., Duchek, J. M., Gernsbacher, M. A., & Smith, S. (1997). Inhibitory control during sentence comprehension in individuals with dementia of the Alzheimer type. *Brain and Language, 57,* 225–253.

Ferrand, L., Segui, J., & Grainger, J. (1996). Masked priming of words and picture naming: The role of syllabic units. *Journal of Memory and Language, 35,* 708–723.

Folstein, M. F., Folstein, S. E., & McHugh, P. R. (1975). "Mini-Mental State": A practical method for grading the cognitive state of patients for the clinician. *Journal of Psychiatric Research*, *12*, 189–198.

Friedman, R. B., Ferguson, S., Robinson, S., & Sunderland, T. (1992). Dissociation of mechanisms of reading in Alzheimer's disease. *Brain and Language*, *43*, 400–413.

Giffard, B., Desgranges, B., Nore-Mary, F., Lalevée, C., de la Sayette, V., & Pasquier, F. et al. (2001). The nature of semantic memory deficits in Alzheimer's disease: New insights from hyperpriming effects. *Brain: A Journal of Neurology*, *124*, 1522–1532.

Hartman, M., & Hasher, L. (1991). Aging and suppression: Memory for previously relevant information. *Psychology and Aging*, *6*, 587–594.

Hasher, L., & Zacks, R. T. (1988). Working memory, comprehension, and aging: A review and a new view. In G. H. Bower (Ed.), *The psychology of learning and motivation*. (Vol. 22, pp. 193–225). New York: Academic Press.

Hasher, L., Zacks, R. T., & Rahhal, T. A. (1999). Timing, instructions, and inhibitory control: Some missing factors in the age and memory debate. *Gerontology*, *45*, 355–357.

Hodges, J. R., Salmon, D. P., & Butters, N. (1992). Semantic memory impairment in Alzheimer's disease: Failure of access or degraded knowledge? *Neuropsychologia*, *30*, 301–314.

Jefferies, E., Patterson, K., Jones, R. W., Bateman, D., & Lambon Ralph, M. A. (2004). A category-specific advantage for numbers in verbal short-term memory: Evidence from semantic dementia. *Neuropsychologia*, *42*, 639–660.

Knott, R., Patterson, K., & Hodges, J. R. (1997). Lexical and semantic binding effects in short-term memory: Evidence from semantic dementia. *Cognitive Neuropsychology*, *14*, 1165–1216.

Margolin, D. I., Pate, D. S., & Friedrich, F. J. (1996). Lexical priming by pictures and words in normal aging and in dementia of the Alzheimer's type. *Brain and Language*, *54*, 275–301.

Mathey, S., & Zagar, D. (2002). Lexical similarity in visual word recognition: The effect of syllabic neighbourhood in French. *Current Psychology Letters: Behavior, Brain & Cognition*, *8*, 107–121.

May, C. P., Zacks, R. T., Hasher, L., & Multhaup, K. S. (1999). Inhibition in the processing of garden-path sentences. *Psychology and Aging*, *14*, 304–313.

McKhann, G., Drachman, D., Folstein, M., Katzman, R., Price, D., & Stadlan, E. M. (1984). Clinical diagnosis of Alzheimer's disease: Report of the NINCDS-ADRDA Work Group under the auspices of Department of Health and Human Services Task Force on Alzheimer's Disease. *Neurology*, *34*, 939–944.

Nebes, R. D. (1992). Semantic memory dysfunction in Alzheimer's disease: Disruption of semantic knowledge or information-processing limitation? In L. R. Squire & N. Butters (Eds.), *Neuropsychology of memory*. (2nd ed., pp. 233–240). New York: Guilford Press.

Nebes, R. D., & Brady, C. B. (1991). The effect of contextual constraint on semantic judgments by Alzheimer patients. *Cortex*, *27*, 237–246.

Nestor, P. J., Scheltens, P., & Hodges, J. R. (2004). Advances in the early detection of Alzheimer's disease. *Nature Medicine*, *10(Suppl)*, 34–41.

Nicholas, M., Obler, L. K., Au, R., & Albert, M. L. (1996). On the nature of naming errors in aging and dementia: A study of semantic relatedness. *Brain and Language*, *54*, 184–195.

Pallier, C., Dupoux, E., & Jeannin, X. (1997). EXPE: An expandable programming language for on-line psychological experiments. *Behavior Research Methods, Instruments, & Computers*, *29*, 322–327.

Patterson, K., Graham, N., & Hodges, J. R. (1994a). Reading in dementia of the Alzheimer type: A preserved ability? *Neuropsychology*, *8*, 395–407.

Patterson, K., Graham, N., & Hodges, J. R. (1994b). The impact of semantic memory loss on phonological representations. *Journal of Cognitive Neuroscience*, *6*, 57–69.

Perea, M., & Carreiras, M. (1998). Effects of syllable frequency and syllable neighbourhood frequency in visual word recognition. *Journal of Experimental Psychology: Human Perception and Performance*, *24*, 134–144.

Perea, M., & Pollatsek, A. (1998). The effects of neighbourhood frequency in reading and lexical decision. *Journal of Experimental Psychology. Human Perception and Performance*, *24*, 767–779.

Rapp, B. (1992). The nature of sublexical orthographic organisation: The bigram trough hypothesis examined. *Journal of Memory and Language*, *31*, 33–53.

Reisberg, B., Ferris, S. H., DeLeon, M. J., & Crook, T. (1982). The global deterioration scale of assessment of primary degenerative dementia. *British Journal of Psychiatry*, *139*, 1136–1139.

Sebastián-Gallés, N., Martí, M. A., Carreiras, M., & Cuetos, F. (2000). *LEXESP: Una base de datos informatizada del español* [*LEXESP: A computerized database of Spanish*]. Universitat de Barcelona, Spain.

Spieler, D. H., Balota, D. A., & Faust, M. E. (1996). Stroop performance in healthy younger and older adults and in individuals with dementia of the Alzheimer's type. *Journal of Experimental Psychology: Human Perception and Performance, 22*, 461–479.

Sullivan, M. P., Faust, M. E., & Balota, D. A. (1995). Identity negative priming in older adults and individuals with dementia of the Alzheimer's type. *Neuropsychology, 9*, 537–555.

Taylor, J. K., & Burke, D. M. (2002). Asymmetric aging effects on semantic and phonological processes: Naming in the picture–word interference task. *Psychology and Aging, 17*, 662.

Woollams, A., Lambon Ralph, M. A., Hodges, J. R., & Patterson, K. (2005). *SD-squared: On the association between semantic dementia and surface dyslexia.* Paper presented at the Experimental Psychology Society conference, Essex, UK.

Zacks, R. T., & Hasher, L. (1994). Directed ignoring: Inhibitory regulation of working memory. In D. Dagenbach & T. H. Carr (Eds.), *Inhibitory mechanisms in attention, memory, and language* (pp. 241–264). New York: Academic Press.

APHASIOLOGY, 2008, 22 (11), 1191–1200

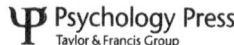

Is there a syllable frequency effect in aphasia or in apraxia of speech or both?

Marina Laganaro

University Hospital, Geneva, Switzerland

Background: The observation of a syllable frequency effect on production latencies in healthy speakers has been an argument in favour of stored syllables in speech production. In Levelt, Roelofs, and Meyer's (1999) model of speech production, syllabic representations are accessed during phonetic encoding. Neurolinguistic studies have provided convergent evidence of a syllable frequency effect on production accuracy in speakers with acquired language disorders. However, the observation that syllable frequency also affected production in aphasic speakers with a pre-phonetic impairment (conduction aphasia and Wernicke's aphasia) seems in contradiction to the phonetic locus of syllabic representations.

Aims: We illustrate the points of convergences and divergences between psycholinguistic and neurolinguistic results on the locus of the syllable frequency effect and explore whether a syllable frequency effect is observed in apraxia of speech (AoS) and in conduction aphasia when participants are tested with the same material.

Methods & Procedures: Reading and repetition was elicited with monosyllabic words (Experiment A) and with bisyllabic pseudowords (Experiment B) composed of high- or low-frequency syllables. Three speakers with AoS and three speakers with conduction aphasia participated in each experiment.

Outcomes & Results: Both subgroups displayed a tendency for a syllable frequency effect on production accuracy. A significant effect of syllable frequency was observed in each experiment in a participant with AoS and in a participant with conduction aphasia.

Conclusions: The data confirmed similar syllable frequency effects in speakers with AoS and in conduction aphasia when tested with the same eliciting material. We discuss these apparently contradictory observations and suggest an explanation for the origin of the syllable frequency effect in these two populations.

Keywords: Language production; Syllable frequency; Phonetic encoding; Phonological encoding; Aphasia; Apraxia of speech.

The syllable is both a very intuitive notion and also, simultaneously, a difficult unit to define precisely. Indeed, every speaker can easily identify or count syllables in a word or in a sentence, because of the perceptual (increasing and decreasing sonority) and functional properties (phonological and poetry rules are applied) of the syllable. By contrast, its exact definition and its role in speech production are still

Address correspondence to: Marina Laganaro, Neurorehabilitation, Geneva University Hospitals, Av. Beau-Séjour 26, CH-1211 Genève 14, Switzerland. E-mail: marina.laganaro@hcuge.ch

I wish to thank Lindsey Nickels and Manuel Carreiras for their meticulous review and helpful comments on a previous version of the manuscript. Research supported by Swiss National Science Foundation Grant No. 105312-108284.

http://www.psypress.com/aphasiology   DOI: 10.1080/02687030701820469

controversial. Two main questions hold research interest about syllables in normal and pathological speech production. The first question is whether syllables are represented and retrieved from a mental store or whether they are computed on-line through phonological rules. The second issue concerns the encoding level at which syllabic information is processed.

These two questions will be illustrated through the presentation of psycholinguistic and neurolinguistic data. We first review the empirical evidence in favour of syllabic representations, and then we focus on the question concerning the locus of syllabic representation. Indeed, most psycholinguistic and neurolinguistic evidence seems to converge concerning the representation of syllables, but some data diverge with regard to the locus of syllable storage and retrieval.

THE REPRESENTATION OF SYLLABLES

The first empirical psycholinguistic evidence concerning the representation of syllables came from the observation that consonants tend to interact with other consonants from homologous syllable positions in slips-of-the-tongue (Shattuck-Hufnagel, 1979). This observation is known as the "syllabic position constraint". However, this observation only proves that abstract syllabic positions are conserved when segments move in slips-of-the-tongue. On the other hand, the fact that slips-of-the-tongue rarely involve surface syllables, has rather been an argument against the representation of phonological syllables. Since our interest here concerns *surface syllables*—that is, the structure *and* the segmental content of the syllable—we will focus only on psycholinguistic and neurolinguistic evidence for surface syllable representation.

The question of syllabic representations has been investigated experimentally with psycholinguistic syllable-priming paradigms, in which researchers tried to speed up the production of words through the presentation of the first syllable of the word (compared to a condition in which the phonological overlap did not correspond to the syllable). These studies led to controversial results. Some authors reported positive syllable-priming effects (Ferrand, Segui, & Grainger, 1996; Ferrand, Segui, & Humphreys, 1997), while other researchers failed to replicate these results, even when the same methods and materials were used (Perret, Bonin, & Méot, 2006; Schiller, 2000; Schiller, Costa, & Colomé, 2002).

An alternative line of investigation has tackled the question of the representation of syllables through the study of syllable *frequency* effects. The underlying idea was that the retrieval of a stored unit should be sensitive to the frequency with which this unit is used. If syllables are explicitly represented, their retrieval can be expected to be a function of their frequency of use. This rationale was introduced by Levelt and Wheeldon (1994) and it has been implemented in both psycholinguistic and in neurolinguistic studies. The initial failure to replicate the syllable frequency effect in speech production (Hendricks & McQueen, 1996; see also Whilshire & Nespoulous, 2002, for a neurolinguistic study) has rapidly been overcome by psycholinguistic and neurolinguistic studies showing a facilitatory effect of syllable frequency on production. Psycholinguistic studies reported shorter production latencies for high-frequency than for low-frequency syllables in several languages (Spanish: Carreiras & Perea, 2004; Perea & Carreiras, 1998; Dutch: Cholin, Levelt, & Schiller, 2006; and French: Laganaro & Alario, 2006). In parallel, neurolinguistic studies have provided evidence for a syllable frequency effect in brain-damaged speakers (Aichert

& Ziegler, 2004; Laganaro, 2005; Stenneken, Hofman, & Jacobs, 2005) with different methodologies and different aphasic profiles.

To sum up, the analysis of the question of syllable representation through the manipulation of syllable frequency led to converging psycholinguistic and neurolinguistic evidence, showing that high-frequency syllables are produced faster and are more resistant to brain damage. Taken together these results argue in favour of the representation and retrieval of syllables rather than their generation by a rule. However, there is a point where the different data do not converge. It concerns the level at which syllables are represented and retrieved during encoding. If psycholinguistic theoretical and experimental data suggest a phonetic origin for the observed syllable frequency effect, some neurolinguistic data seem not to converge with the interpretation of phonetic syllables. Indeed, the syllable frequency effect has been reported with brain-damaged speakers whose impairment is thought to affect different levels of encoding: patients with apraxia of speech (Aichert & Ziegler, 2004; Staiger & Ziegler, 2008 this issue), conduction aphasia (Laganaro, 2005), and Wernicke's aphasia (Stenneken et al., 2005).

THE LOCUS OF SYLLABLE REPRESENTATION

A current model of speech production (Levelt et al., 1999) includes syllabic representations at the level of phonetic encoding. The level of phonetic encoding constitutes the interface between phonological encoding and articulation. Syllable representations in the form of syllabic gestural scores are accessed in this model during phonetic encoding to build up the phonetic form of the phonological word to be produced. There are no phonological representations of syllables according to this model—only earlier and discontinued versions of Dell's connectionist model (Dell, 1986) included stored syllable units at the phonological level. The evidence in favour of phonetic syllables rather than phonological syllables is based on linguistic data and on experimental studies. First, the resyllabification of sequences across "deep" syllable boundaries in connected speech production has been an argument against stored phonological syllables (for example, in a sequence like cher ami – "dear friend" – the syllabic structure of the surface form [Sɛ.Ra.mi– CV.CV.CV – is different from that of the individual forms [SɛR] – CVC – and [ami] – V.CV).

While the experimental paradigms of previous psycholinguistic studies reporting a syllable frequency effect did not allow differentiation of a phonological from a phonetic effect, Laganaro and Alario (2006) reported evidence in favour of a phonetic locus of the syllable frequency effect with a delayed production paradigm. In this study the facilitatory syllable frequency effect on production latencies survived in delayed production only when the delay was filled with an articulatory suppression task. As articulatory suppression is thought to prevent phonetic encoding, the results suggested a phonetic locus of the syllable frequency effect.

If stored syllables are represented and retrieved during phonetic encoding, neurolinguistic evidence for a syllable frequency effect should be observed in apraxia of speech, since its cause is thought to be impaired phonetic encoding (Blumstein, 1990; Code, 1998; Darley, Aronson, & Brown, 1975; Varley & Whiteside, 2001). Among the neurolinguistic reports of syllable frequency effects, only the data by Aichert and Ziegler (2004) and by Staiger and Ziegler (2008 this issue) are in line with a phonetic repository of syllables, since the effect was observed with speakers with apraxia of speech (AoS). The observations of a syllable frequency effect on accuracy and on the substitution errors of patients with conduction aphasia (Laganaro, 2005) and in the distribution of a jargon-aphasic patient's neologisms (Stenneken et al., 2005) seem in contradiction with a phonetic interpretation of the effect. Indeed, the locus of impairment is phonological rather than phonetic in those patients.

In the experimental study with AoS speakers (Aichert & Ziegler, 2004) the frequency of the first syllable was manipulated in disyllabic German words, and AoS speakers were more impaired when producing the words containing the low-frequency syllables than those with the high-frequency syllables. In the study with conduction aphasia, the syllable frequency effect has been reported on substitution errors and on non-word repetition in Italian, French, and Spanish (Laganaro, 2005). Phoneme substitution errors were found to generate syllables of higher frequency than the target syllables in three participants with conduction aphasia; three other participants produced fewer errors on non-words composed of high-frequency syllables than on non-words composed of low-frequency syllables. Finally, in the study with a Wernicke's aphasic speaker, a syllable frequency effect was observed in the distributional analysis of German neologistic utterances (Stenneken et al., 2005). The produced syllables were of higher frequency than the normal German syllable frequency distribution, indicating that the aphasic participant was producing a high proportion of frequent syllables.

In sum, evidence for syllable frequency effects in different aphasic profiles comes from different languages or from different eliciting material and analyses. In order to clarify whether the same effect is really observed with different kinds of impairment, we report data from a study using the same eliciting material with AoS and with conduction aphasia.

EXPERIMENT A: MONOSYLLABIC WORDS

In this study we analysed the effect of syllable frequency on production accuracy in participants with AoS and with conduction aphasia. Monosyllabic words were used in this experiment because they allow syllable frequency to be easily manipulated while controlling for lexical frequency and syllable structure.

Method

Materials. A total of 60 French monosyllabic words were selected. Half of the words corresponded to low-frequency syllables and half to high-frequency syllables. Low-frequency syllables (for example: *chaud* [So] – hot, *clou* ([klu] – nail) had token occurrences below 260 per million in the BRULEX database (Content, Mousty, & Radeau, 1996) syllabified in Goslin and Frauenfelder (2000) (range: 2–259). High-frequency syllables (example: *dé* [de] – dice; *trou* [tRu] – hole) had occurrences above 360 (range 364–13000). The two syllable frequency groups were matched pairwise on CV structure and did not differ significantly on lexical frequency, $t(58) = 1.67$, $p = .1$.

Procedure. All the participants performed a repetition and a reading task during different sessions. Words were presented verbally or visually in a pseudo-randomised order and participants were asked to repeat or to read them aloud. Each participant's production was transcribed on-line by the experimenter and tape-recorded for verification.

Participants. Three speakers presenting with conduction aphasia and three speakers with apraxia of speech took part in the study. They were native French speakers and had impaired production even for monosyllabic words. Their demographic information is given in Table 1. The participants were classified by at least two speech and language therapists as conduction aphasic or AoS on the basis of classical classification criteria. To be classified as AoS, the production had to be characterised by non-fluent speech with syllabification (intersyllabic pauses) or initiation difficulties such as groping, and the segmental errors had to include a high proportion of single feature transformations (especially voicing or articulatory position) or of distorted phonemes. The conduction aphasic participants had fluent speech characterised by phonological transformations, including neologisms and *conduites d'approche*, which had to be observed in all verbal output modalities (spontaneous, naming, reading, and repetition). Patients CA1 and CA2 had conduction aphasia associated with agraphia; CA3 has evolved from initial Wernicke's aphasia to conduction aphasia and produced many neologisms. Among the AoS patients, AoS2 presented with Broca's aphasia associated with apraxia of speech; AoS1 had apraxia of speech with very mild agraphia; AoS3 did not display oral or written language impairments, but had apraxia of speech associated to a mild dysarthria.

Results

Only productions that were entirely correct at first attempt were scored as correct. Individual scores for high- and low-frequency syllables are shown in Table 2.

Production accuracy was higher for high-frequency than for low-frequency monosyllabic words in four out of six participants. The syllable frequency effect was significant for one participant with conduction aphasia (CA2) on the total score and one participant with AoS (AoS2) on repetition. One participant from each subgroup had similar production accuracy on low and on high syllable frequency monosyllabic words.

An interim conclusion from these results is that conduction aphasia and AoS speakers do not differ on production accuracy on monosyllabic words composed of high and low syllable frequency. A significant syllable frequency effect was observed

TABLE 1
Demographic data for the participants of Experiment A

	Aphasia sub-type	Aetiology and lesion	Months post-onset	Age
CA1	Conduction aphasia	CVA, left insular and parietal	9	62
CA2	Conduction aphasia	Left fronto-temporal-parietal contusion	7	50
CA3	Conduction aphasia	CVA, left parietal	2	81
AoS1	Apraxia of speech	CVA, Left anterior with left fronto- opercular	2	52
AoS2	Broca aphasia	CVA, Left capsulo-lenticular and fronto-temporal	2	39
AoS3	Apraxia of speech	CVA Left temporal	2	50

TABLE 2
Percent correct production for high- and low-frequency syllables and significant p values at
Fisher's exact test

	Total			Repetition			Reading	
	low Syll-F	high Syll-F	Fisher's p	low Syll-F	high Syll-F	Fisher's p	low Syll- F	high Syll- F
CA1	42%	40%		43%	43%		42%	40%
CA2	30%	50%	0.04	40%	67%	0.07	10%	17%
CA3	67%	73%		70%	87%		63%	60%
AoS1	88%	87%		87%	83%		90%	90%
AoS2	62%	78%	0.07	40%	70%	0.04	83%	87%
AoS3	60%	67%		70%	73%		50%	60%

for one participant from each subgroup. The other participants had a tendency for better performance with high-frequency syllables.

Before any further interpretation, we analysed whether a similar pattern of results is observed with a different production task. In the following experiment a non-word material was used, which had the advantage that other possible confounds, such as phoneme frequency, could also be controlled for.

EXPERIMENT B: DISYLLABIC PSEUDOWORDS

Method

Materials. We created 40 bisyllabic pseudowords. Half of the pseudowords were composed of two low-frequency syllables (sum of occurrences below 159 per million in the BRULEX database; examples: [givõ], [nyʀsak]) and 20 bisyllabic pseudowords were composed of two high-frequency syllables (sum of frequencies above 300 occurrences per million; examples: [gyʃo], [naldãs]). High and low syllable frequency pseudowords were matched pairwise on the CV structure of both syllables and did not significantly differ on phoneme frequency, $t(38) < 1$. For the reading task, an orthographic transcription was found for each pseudoword by using the most frequent French phoneme-to-grapheme conversion while controlling for the number of graphemes across the two syllable frequency groups.

Procedure. All the participants performed a repetition and a reading task during different sessions. Five participants performed each task twice. The stimuli were presented verbally or visually by DmDX software (Forster & Forster, 2003) and participants were asked to repeat or to read each pseudoword without time pressure. Participants were seated in front of the computer screen and wore a head-mounted microphone. After explaining the task with the help of some training trials, participants went through the task alone in a quiet room. The spoken responses were digitised within 5 seconds after the end of the spoken stimuli or from the moment the visual stimulus appeared on the screen.

Participants. Three participants with conduction aphasia and three participants with apraxia of speech took part in Experiment B. Three participants from

Experiment A, who could read and repeat correctly some disyllabic pseudowords, also participated in this experiment (CA3, AoS1, and AoS3). For the other participants the selecting criteria were the same as for Experiment A. Participant CA4 presented conduction aphasia with alexia and agraphia; CA5 had mild conduction aphasia; and AoS4 had apraxia of speech associated with a mild dysgraphia. Their demographic data are given in Table 3.

Results

Only productions that were entirely correct at the first attempt were scored as correct. Results showed better performance with pseudowords composed of high-frequency syllables in all participants (see Table 4).

The syllable frequency effect reached significance in one participant with conduction aphasia (CA3) and in one participant with apraxia of speech (AoS1). In each case the significant total score was due more to the repetition task than to performance on the reading task.

It should be noted that neither participant CA3 nor AoS1 displayed a syllable frequency effect in Experiment A, probably because of their scores being close to ceiling in the monosyllabic word production task.

Overall, these results replicate those of Experiment A, indicating similar patterns in the subgroup of participants with apraxia of speech and in the subgroup with conduction aphasia. Moreover, these results allow us to exclude an interference of

TABLE 3
Demographic data for the participants of Experiment B

	Aphasia sub-type	Aetiology, lesion	Months post-onset	Age
CA4	Conduction aphasia	CVA, left temporo-parieto-occipital	10	57
CA5	Conduction aphasia	CVA, left temporal	1	59
AoS4	Apraxia of speech	CVA, left fronto-opercular	3	53

TABLE 4
Percent correct production for high and low syllable frequency non-words and significant
p values at Fisher's exact test

	Total			Repetition			Reading	
	Low-frequency syllables	High-frequency syllables	Fisher's p	Low-frequency syllables	High-frequency syllables	Fisher's p	Low-frequency syllables	High-frequency syllables
CA3	19%	35%	*0.03*	8%	28%	*0.04*	30%	43%
CA4**	40%	58%		40%	58%		.	
CA5	61%	71%		73%	78%		50%	65%
AoS1	46%	68%	*0.01*	50%	73%	0.06	43%	63%
AoS3	39%	45%		50%	48%		28%	43%
AoS4*	55%	58%		80%	75%		25%	40%

*Reading and repetition was elicited only once. ** Reading was not analysed because of very impaired pseudoword reading.

phoneme frequency on the observed syllable frequency effect, since phoneme frequency was balanced across the two syllable frequency conditions.

DISCUSSION AND CONCLUSION

Taken together, results from Experiments A and B indicate similar patterns of results in the subgroup of participants with AoS and in the subgroups of conduction aphasia. Individuals from both subgroups displayed a tendency for a syllable frequency effect on production accuracy. A significant effect of syllable frequency was observed in two participants with conduction aphasia and in two speakers with AoS. These results confirm that the effects reported in the neurolinguistic literature by different research groups with AoS participants and with aphasic participants presenting phonological impairment are not due to the bias of using different languages and different methodologies. Also, as already reported in previous studies (Aichert & Ziegler, 2004; Laganaro, 2005), the effect was not observed in all participants, since at least one participant from each subgroup was not affected by syllable frequency. The present results suggest that severity of impairment and difficulty of the eliciting material may at least partially explain these observations. Indeed, two participants who did not display a syllable frequency effect in Experiment A, and who had high production accuracy with the material of that experiment, were affected by syllable frequency in Experiment B, where they were more impaired.

In both experiments the syllable frequency effect was more robust in repetition than in reading aloud. This observation may suggest that input processes play a role in the observed effect. However, we can rule out an explanation based entirely on perceptive effects, because a trend for a syllable frequency effect appeared in the reading task for most participants, especially in Experiment B, and because the same effects have been reported in studies using other eliciting methods (see the introduction). The observed syllable frequency effect is probably a production effect, but an additional input effect may have emerged in the repetition task or a confound factor may have interfered with syllable frequency in the reading task.

The observation that participants with apraxia of speech and with conduction aphasia display a similar syllable frequency effect on production accuracy challenges the interpretation of the locus of this effect or of the underlying locus of impairment in these two subgroups. We have presented in the introduction an overview of the arguments in favour of a phonetic locus of the syllable frequency effect. The hypothesis that syllables are stored and retrieved in order to build the phonetic plan of an utterance to be produced is in line with the observation that brain-damaged patients with an impaired phonetic encoding (AoS) show a syllable frequency effect. In these patients, high-frequency syllables are more resistant to the damage and are more easily produced. By contrast, it is more difficult to reconcile the syllable frequency effect observed in participants with conduction aphasia (and in those with Wernicke's aphasia, see Stenneken et al., 2005), whose impairment is thought to touch a pre-phonetic encoding stage. These results need to be discussed, because they seem at odds with a phonetic representation of syllables.

The observation that speakers with impaired phonological encoding are affected by syllable frequency may be interpreted as an evidence for stored phonological syllables, as in the earlier version of Dell's model of phonological encoding (Dell, 1986). However, if the hypothesis of stored phonological syllables is ruled out in accordance with the arguments presented in the introduction, an alternative explanation should be found.

In Laganaro (2005) we suggested that the syllable frequency effect observed in the substitution errors of speakers with conduction aphasia may be due to the default retrieval of more frequent syllables from an incomplete phonological input. This means that a phonological impairment leads in some cases to an incomplete or underspecified phonological representation, and that syllables of high frequency are addressed by default when some phonological information is missing. A similar mechanism called "phonological reconstruction" had already been suggested by Kohn and Smith (1994) and by Butterworth (1992). This mechanism attributes by default phonological information when it is missing due to damage to phonological encoding. It makes sense to assume that "phonological reconstruction" selects the most available representation; for instance, the more frequent syllables. This explanation of a default retrieval of high-frequency syllables is in line with both the phonetic locus of syllables and the phonological level of impairment in conduction aphasia. However, the default retrieval of high-frequency syllables fits better with the observation that the produced syllables are of higher frequency than the targeted syllables, than with better performance on words or non-words composed of high-frequency syllables. Indeed, how can we explain the fact that the manipulation of syllable frequency in the eliciting material also affects the correct production in cases with pre-phonetic impairment? If we rule out the hypothesis of phonological syllables, the fact that the frequency of phonetic syllables affects production accuracy in aphasic speakers with a pre-phonetic locus of impairment suggests an interaction between the two levels of encoding. Feedback activation from phonetic syllables to the level of phonological encoding may facilitate the encoding of phonological information linked to high-frequency syllables, especially when phonological encoding is impaired. This suggestion may account for the syllable frequency effect observed in the subgroup of conduction aphasia but this issue needs further empirical verification.

In conclusion, the observation of a similar effect of syllable frequency in apraxia of speech and in conduction aphasia seems contradictory, because of different underlying impairments, but may be explained by different mechanisms—defective encoding of low-frequency syllables in the case of phonetic impairment and default attribution of frequent syllables, or feedback effects from the syllabary to phonological encoding in cases with pre-phonetic impairment.

REFERENCES

Aichert, I., & Ziegler, W. (2004). Syllable frequency and syllable structure in apraxia of speech. *Brain and Language, 88*, 148–159.

Blumstein, S. (1990). Phonological deficits in aphasia: Theoretical perspectives. In A. Caramazza (Ed.), *Cognitive neuropsychology and neurolinguistics* (pp. 33–53). Hillsdale, NJ: Lawrence Erlbaum Associates Inc.

Butterworth, B. (1992). Disorders of phonological encoding. *Cognition, 42*, 261–286.

Carreiras, M., & Perea, M. (2004). Naming pseudowords in Spanish: Effects of syllable frequency. *Brain and Language, 90*, 393–400.

Cholin, J., Levelt, W. J. M., & Schiller, N. O. (2006). Effects of syllable frequency in speech production. *Cognition, 99*, 205–235.

Code, C. (1998). Major review: Models, theories and heuristics in apraxia of speech. *Clinical Linguistics and Phonetics, 12,* 47–65.

Content, A., Mousty, P., & Radeau, M. (1990). Brulex. Une base de données lexicales informatisées pour le français écrit & parlé. *L'Année Psychologique, 90,* 551–566.

Darley, F., Aronson, A., & Brown, J. (1975). *Motor speech disorders.* Philadelphia: W. B. Saunders.

Dell, G. S. (1986). A spreading-activation theory of retrieval in sentence production. *Psychological Review, 9,* 283–321.

Ferrand, L., Segui, J., & Grainger, J. (1996). Masked priming of word and picture naming: The role of syllabic units. *Journal of Memory and Language, 35,* 708–723.

Ferrand, L., Segui, J. S., & Humphreys, G. W. (1997). The syllable's role in word naming. *Memory and Cognition, 25,* 458–470.

Forster, K. I., & Forster, J. C. (2003). DMDX: A windows display program with millisecond accuracy. *Behavior Research Methods, Instruments & Computers, 35,* 116–124.

Kohn, S. E., & Smith, K. L. (1994). Distinction between two phonological output deficits. *Applied psycholinguistics, 15,* 75–95.

Goslin, J., & Frauenfelder, U. H. (2000). A comparison of theoretical and human syllabification. *Language and Speech, 44,* 409–436.

Hendricks, H., & McQueen, J. (Eds.). (1996). *Max Planck Institute for Psycholinguistics, Annual Report 1995.* Nijmegen: Max Planck Institute for Psycholinguistics.

Laganaro, M. (2005). Syllable frequency effect in speech production: Evidence from aphasia. *Journal of Neurolinguistics, 18,* 221–235.

Laganaro, M., & Alario, F. X. (2006). On the locus of syllable frequency effect. *Journal of Memory and Language, 55,* 178–196.

Levelt, W. J. M., Roelofs, A., & Meyer, A. S. (1999). A theory of lexical access in speech production. *Behavioral and Brain Sciences, 22,* 1–75.

Levelt, W. J. M., & Wheeldon, L. (1994). Do speakers have access to mental syllabary? *Cognition, 50,* 289–269.

Perea, M., & Carreiras, M. (1998). Effects of syllable frequency and syllable neighbourhood frequency in visual word recognition. *Journal of Experimental Psychology: Human Perception and Performance, 24,* 134–144.

Perret, C., Bonin, P., & Méot, A. (2006). Syllable priming effects in picture naming in French: Lost in the sea! *Experimental Psychology, 53,* 95–104.

Schiller, N. O. (2000). Single word production in English: The role of subsyllabic units during phonological encoding. *Journal of Experimental Psychology: Learning Memory and Cognition, 26,* 512–528.

Schiller, N. O., Costa, A., & Colomé, A. (2002). Phonological encoding of single words: In search of the lost syllable. In C. Gussenhoven & N. Warner (Eds.), *Laboratory phonology VII* (pp. 35–59). Berlin: Mouton de Gruyter.

Shattuck-Hufnagel, S. (1979). Speech errors as evidence for a serial order mechanism in sentence production. In W. E. Cooper & E. C. Walker (Eds.), *Sentence processing* (pp. 295–342). Hillsdale, NJ: Lawrence Erlbaum Associates Inc.

Staiger, A., & Ziegler, W. (2008). Syllable frequency and syllable structure in the spontaneous speech production of patients with apraxia of speech. *Aphasiology, 22,* 1201–1215.

Stenneken, P., Hofman, M., & Jacobs, A. M. (2005). Patterns of phoneme and syllable frequency in jargon aphasia. *Brain and Language, 95,* 221–222.

Varley, R., & Whiteside, S. (2001). What is the underlying impairment in acquired apraxia of speech? *Aphasiology, 15,* 39–49.

Whilshire, C. E., & Nespoulous, J. L. (2002). Syllables as units in speech production: Data from aphasia. *Brain and Language, 84,* 424–447.

APHASIOLOGY, 2008, 22 (11), 1201–1215

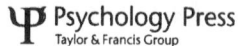

Syllable frequency and syllable structure in the spontaneous speech production of patients with apraxia of speech

Anja Staiger and Wolfram Ziegler

EKN – Clinical Neuropsychology Research Group, München, Germany

Background: The sublexical factors syllable frequency and syllable structure are known to influence error rates in patients with apraxia of speech (e.g., Aichert & Ziegler, 2004; Romani & Galluzzi, 2005). To our knowledge, these factors have almost exclusively been examined by single-word production paradigms. However, performance on single-word tasks is not necessarily a good predictor of spontaneous speech production, since the generation of conversational speech involves specific conditions and additional demands. This might influence the weights of syllable frequency and syllable structure in explanations of the accuracy of speech production in apraxic speakers.
Aims: Our aim was to determine if the spontaneous speech production of patients with apraxia of speech (AOS) is influenced by the factors syllable frequency and syllable structure. The two research questions that guided our investigation were: (1) Are the distribution properties of syllables in spontaneous speech different in patients with AOS compared to unimpaired speakers? (2) Do the factors syllable frequency and syllable structure affect articulatory accuracy in the spontaneous speech of patients with AOS?
Methods & Procedures: Three patients with AOS and 15 neurologically unimpaired control persons produced samples of spontaneous speech with a minimum of 1000 syllables each. Structure and frequency counts were made on the basis of the German CELEX database.
Outcomes & Results: The distribution properties of the spontaneous speech samples were similar in the apraxic speakers and the unimpaired controls. In all three patients the proportion of errors was significantly higher on low- than on high-frequency syllables. In two patients a significant effect even persisted when any confound with syllable structure was ruled out. Syllable structure effects were only found within the low-frequency syllables.
Conclusions: Syllable frequency and syllable structure play a decisive role with respect to articulatory accuracy in the spontaneous speech production of patients with AOS.

Keywords: Spontaneous speech production; Apraxia of speech; Syllable frequency; Syllable structure.

A widely accepted definition proposed by Darley, Aronson, and Brown (1975) describes apraxia of speech (AOS) as an "articulatory disorder resulting from impairment due to brain damage of the capacity to program the positioning of

Address correspondence to: Anja Staiger, EKN – Clinical Neuropsychology Research Group, Dachauerstr. 164, 80992 München, Germany. E-mail: anja.staiger@extern.lrz-muenchen.de

The first author of this study was supported by a grant from the DFG - German research council (ZI 469/10-2). We would also like to thank the ReHa-Hilfe e.V. for their support. We are grateful to our colleagues from the Neuropsychological Clinic, Munich-Bogenhausen Hospital, Munich, and to the staff from the speech therapy departments at the Rehabilitation Hospitals Bad Heilbrunn and Bad Aibling for their collaboration on clinical issues. We would also like to express our gratitude to all participants.

http://www.psypress.com/aphasiology   DOI: 10.1080/02687030701820584

speech musculature for the volitional production of phonemes and the sequencing of muscle movements" (p. 255). In reference to models of speech production, AOS can be attributed to the phonetic encoding level (Code, 1998; Nickels & Howard, 2000; Varley & Whiteside, 2001; Ziegler, 2002). As a phonetic encoding deficit, AOS is distinguished from impairments of phonological encoding processes (i.e., aphasia) as well as from deficits affecting the articulatory network (i.e., dysarthria).

It is assumed that during phonetic encoding speakers access a store of holistic articulatory-phonetic programmes for the frequently occurring syllables of a particular language, the so-called *mental syllabary* (Levelt, Roelofs, & Meyer, 1999). By contrast, the articulatory plans for new or very low-frequency syllables are not retrieved from the mental syllabary but assembled from smaller units. The postulate of a mental syllabary is motivated by results showing that the production of high-frequency syllables involves shorter naming latencies than the production of syllables with lower frequencies (Carreiras & Perea, 2004; Cholin, 2008 this issue; Cholin, Levelt, & Schiller, 2006; Levelt & Wheeldon, 1994; see also Laganaro & Alario, 2006).

As the syllable appears to be a relevant unit in the process of phonetic encoding, investigations of parameters relating to the syllable may also throw light on the pathomechanisms underlying AOS. Aichert and Ziegler (2004) examined whether patients with AOS still have access to the mental syllabary. From their finding of an influence of syllable frequency on the occurrence of errors in speakers with AOS, two conclusions can be drawn: First, the observed effects show that these patients do have access to the precompiled gestural scores for syllables in the mental syllabary, but that the units stored there are (at least partially) damaged. Thus, these findings are incompatible with a claim raised by Varley and Whiteside (2001), who postulated a subsyllabic encoding mechanism in AOS. Second, the fact that high-frequency syllables were relatively better preserved than low-frequency syllables suggests a frequency-based organisation of the mental syllabary. Although these results fit neatly into the concept of a phonetic encoding deficit, Laganaro (2005) demonstrated similar effects in patients with aphasic-phonological impairments (see also Laganaro, 2008 this issue).

As another factor influencing the accuracy of speech production in patients with AOS, articulatory complexity has frequently been reported. Patients make more errors on increasingly complex speech units and they tend to systematically replace complex units by less complex ones (e.g., consonant clusters by singletons). Many authors (e.g., Canter, Trost, & Burns, 1985; Nespoulous, Joanette, Beland, Caplan, & Lecours, 1984; Rosenbek, Kent, & La Pointe, 1984; Trost & Canter, 1974) define articulatory complexity as a property of linearly ordered segment strings, considering any sequence of two consonants as complex irrespective of its position within a syllable or across a syllable boundary. However, Aichert and Ziegler (2004) found that the error susceptibility of a consonant cluster is related to its position within a syllable (i.e., in onset vs coda position) or across a syllable boundary, respectively. Following theoretical frameworks that incorporate the syllable as representational unit, complexity of syllable structure has been emphasised and largely confirmed as an influencing factor. Some authors (e.g., Romani & Calabrese, 1998; Romani & Galluzzi, 2005) referred to a complexity measure that scales the syllable templates on a markedness continuum, with any deviation from the simple CV syllable being considered a complication (Clements & Keyser, 1983). Other accounts were based on complexity concepts defined in terms of "number of intra-syllabic clusters" (Nickels & Howard, 2004; Romani & Galluzzi, 2005). A relationship that needs to be kept in mind, however, is that complex syllables tend to be less frequent than simple syllables, so that the two factors—syllable frequency and syllable structure—are confounded.

The above results are, like much of our knowledge about error mechanisms in AOS, based on single-word production experiments (e.g., naming or repetition of single words). Although single-word paradigms offer great advantages (e.g., stimulus control), they imply clear disadvantages as well. Apart from constituting an artificial condition, the results from single-word studies do not allow for safe inferences regarding natural, spontaneous speech production. For example, speech error analyses based on data from normal speakers revealed that *context* strongly influences the occurrence of slips in natural speech (Shattuck-Hufnagel, 1992; Stemberger & Treiman, 1986; Stemberger 1990, 1991). Such interaction errors (occurring between adjacent words) include exchanges, anticipations, and perseverations.

Even though no direct inferences can be drawn from normal slips to the error mechanisms in patients with neurological speech and language disorders, Kohn and Smith (1990) reported on "between-word" errors in a conduction aphasic patient, which resembled the contextually driven errors of normal speakers. Therefore, potential contextual influences on the error patterns of aphasic or apraxic patients should not be neglected. They might even lead to shifts in the weights of the parameters of syllable frequency and syllable structure in explanations of the accuracy of production of these speakers.

Furthermore, it cannot be ruled out that modifications of the above findings emerge due to another noteworthy property of the production of connected speech, i.e., the frequent occurrence of phrase-level phonetic processes. These processes cause deviations from canonical word forms, such as segmental assimilation and elision (e.g., [oːbən] > [oːbn] > [oːbm], Engl. "above"; Kohler, 1990, 2001). Thus, irrespective of the specific phonetic-phonological skills that are required to realise these processes, sentence-level phonetic-phonological rule applications are observed as resulting in changes of the structures of spoken syllables, often involving structural complications (Schiller, 1997).

For these reasons, the present study is an attempt—the first, to our knowledge— to examine the role of syllabic properties on the accuracy of spontaneously produced connected speech in patients with AOS. Such an attempt encounters a number of challenges, a major problem resulting from the fact that examinations of free speech allow no a priori expectations on the linguistic properties of the utterances a speaker is going to produce. In order to guarantee that the major factors influencing the errors can be disentangled, a large data corpus must therefore be collected from each patient. Furthermore, the fact that in spontaneous speech different speakers produce different materials impedes a group-wise pooling of the data.

In the following, speech samples from three apraxic patients elicited in an interview and in a narration task were examined. We carefully selected patients with only mild to moderate AOS and no or minor aphasic impairment. The speech samples were analysed on two coarse analysis levels: First, they were scrutinised for distribution properties of syllable frequencies and syllable structures. Second, an error analysis was undertaken to find out if articulatory accuracy in patients with AOS was influenced by the same factors as in single-word tasks, i.e., frequency and structure of syllabic units.

METHOD

Participants

Three patients with a primary diagnosis of apraxia of speech (AOS) and 15 neurologically healthy individuals participated in the study. All participants were native speakers of German with no or only mild regional accents.

We explicitly selected patients with a clear picture of AOS, little or no concomitant aphasic impairment, and the ability to produce substantial samples of connected speech with a high proportion of intelligible speech units.

The selection of patients was first guided by the clinical judgements of experienced speech and language pathologists. The presence of AOS was further scrutinised on the basis of a repetition test ("Hierarchische Wortlisten – Repetition test for the diagnostic investigation of apraxia of speech"; Liepold, Ziegler, & Brendel, 2003) and of spontaneous speech samples. The results of the repetition test are outlined in Table 1. AOS was diagnosed following criteria that included the occurrence of phonemic and phonetic errors, disturbances at the suprasegmental level (e.g., syllable segregation, dysfluencies), speech initiation difficulties, visible and audible groping, as well as increased speech effort. These criteria were met in the participating patients (see below) and there was an agreement between the clinicians' diagnoses and the first author's judgements in all cases. Moreover, the diagnoses were confirmed independently by two further experienced neurolinguists. In the following, the characteristics of each patient are described in further detail.

Patient RK, a 49-year-old engineer, suffered an ischaemic CVA of the left middle cerebral artery after an intracardiac catheter examination. He was examined 1 month post onset. The patient's speech production was characterised by frequent phonetic and phonemic errors, which occurred inconsistently and were often followed by self-corrections. On the suprasegmental level RK exhibited a disfluent, monotone manner of speaking. This impression was, among others, due to a pattern of syllable segregation. Furthermore, the patient exhibited articulatory groping behaviour as

TABLE 1
Description of participants with apraxia of speech (AOS)

	RK	FL	KH
Age	49	49	65
Gender	m	m	f
Aetiology	ischaemic CVA (mca, left)	ischaemic CVA (mca, left)	ischaemic CVA (mca, left)
Time post onset (months)	1	36	1
AOS severity score	mild-moderate	mild-moderate	mild-moderate
HWL-score[a]:			
Phonemically distorted words	22/96	20/96	37/96
Phonetically distorted words	29/96	25/96	26/96
Dysfluencies	38/96	14/96	28/96
Aphasia type	no aphasia *	mild anomic aphasia*	no aphasia **

[a]Hierarchische Wortlisten – Repetition test for the diagnostic investigation of Apraxia of Speech; Liepold et al., 2003); * based on AAT; ** based on AAT screening (Token Test, Written Language subtest).

well as a noticeable speech effort. Patient RK was diagnosed with a pure, mild to moderate AOS. An aphasic pathology could be ruled out by the Aachener Aphasie Test (AAT; Huber, Poeck, Weniger, & Willmes, 1983).

Patient FL, a 49-year-old cook, suffered an ischaemic CVA of the left middle cerebral artery. He was examined 36 months post onset. FL produced many phonetic and phonemic speech errors, which occurred inconsistently. His speech approached normal fluency and was characterised by a relatively natural prosodic structure, but was nonetheless frequently interrupted by self-corrections, pauses, and sound prolongations. Hardly any visible groping or obvious speech effort could be detected. Patient FL was diagnosed as having a mild to moderate AOS and a concomitant mild aphasic component which mainly affected word retrieval (AAT; Huber et al., 1983). Additionally, FL showed minimal perceptual symptoms of a persisting dysarthria.

Patient KH, a 65-year-old retired cook and housewife, suffered an ischaemic CVA of the left middle cerebral artery. She was examined approximately 1 month post onset. KH's speech production was characterised by a substantial number of phonetic and phonemic errors, which occurred with no apparent consistency. The patient's speech appeared to be reasonably fluent but with some scanning speech rhythm and hesitations, associated particularly with articulatory groping and self-corrections. The speech lacked pronounced speech effort. KH was diagnosed as having mild to moderate AOS. Selected subtests of the AAT (Huber et al., 1983), revealed no aphasia. Nevertheless, due to slight word-finding difficulties and a mild agrammatism, which occurred in connected speech production, as well as to mild impairments in reading comprehension, a residual aphasic component was considered. The descriptive data of the patients are outlined in Table 1.

The control group consisted of 6 male and 9 female neurologically healthy persons with an average age of 41 (range: 21–63).

Procedure

All participants were examined under the same experimental conditions. To collect samples of spontaneous speech we arranged an interview with questions about three everyday life topics, i.e., profession, vacation, and weekend activities. Second, we requested that the participants retell the storyline from a film they had seen lately, as well as from two short video (cartoon) sequences. All speech samples were recorded on audio and video tape (microphone: beyerdynamic TG-X-58, video camera: Panasonic NV-GS180). The samples contained a minimum of 1000 syllables per participant (mean controls: 1701, range: 1029–3091; RK: 1171, FL: 1640, KH: 1170). Analyses were conducted using both the auditory and the visual (mouth movement) information.

The analysis of the raw speech data was carried out in several steps. We first transcribed the speech samples using IPA broad phonetic transcription (with phonetically distorted units being marked by diacritics). These transcripts represented the actually realised utterances produced by the participants.

Starting from these realised forms, the transcripts had to be revised, i.e., we reconstructed the respective canonical forms (or citation forms), stored in lexical databases. More precisely, as canonical forms we considered (1) words that were correct with respect to their phonological form (i.e., phonologically erroneous words were revised), (2) words that were cleared from all phonetic-phonological changes permitted to occur at phrase level (e.g., assimilations, elisions). We also assigned parts of words (e.g., false starts) to their analogous "canonical word parts" as long as they reached syllable size. However, we were only able to assign utterances that unequivocally corresponded to recognisable lexical units. Speech segments (syllables, words, or indefinite units) that were unrecognisable, e.g., due to technical artefacts or unintelligible speech, were excluded from further analyses. The numbers of excluded speech segments were 20 for RK, 66 for FL, and 87 for KH.

The canonical words were then parsed into syllables. The syllables were analysed with respect to their frequency as represented by the syllable rank, with rank 1 corresponding to the most frequent syllable. Next, the structure for each syllable was assigned. Syllables that contained at least one consonant cluster were counted as "complex". For the purpose of these analyses, we used the "Software for Material Analysis and Construction" (Aichert, Marquardt & Ziegler, 2007b). This software operates on the "German Database for Sublexical Frequencies and Structures" (Aichert, Marquardt & Ziegler, 2007a) derived from the CELEX database (Baayen, Piepenbrock, & Gulickers, 1995).

Finally, error analyses of the speech data were carried out for each patient. The evaluation of errors was in turn related to the canonical syllables and restricted to segmental speech errors, i.e., phonemic errors and phonetic distortions. As phonemic errors we counted substitutions, omissions, and additions. Both non-contextual and contextual errors were included into the analyses. The number and position of errors within a syllable was not considered here.

RESULTS

Distribution properties of the spontaneous speech samples

In order to detect if deviant patterns (e.g., more high-frequency syllables or less complex forms) occurred in the patients, we first examined the distribution properties of the spontaneous speech samples of all participants. Analyses included the Type–Token Ratio and the distribution of structure- and frequency-related properties. For this purpose, the canonical forms were considered. Iterations and initiation difficulties such as false starts or articulatory groping were omitted from the analysis. Syllables that could not be attributed unequivocally to a canonical syllable were discarded. The sample of syllables thus obtained comprised a minimum of 1000 per participant.

Type–Token ratio. The Type–Token ratio (TT ratio) measures the proportion of syllable types per syllable token. Figure 1 shows the TT ratio for each participant as a function of the total number of syllable tokens produced. Regarding the healthy control persons, the TT ratio turned out to show a remarkable variability, which was related to the quantity of syllable units produced: the ratio declined as the number of tokens increased. This indicates that participants who talked more did not also produce substantially more syllable types, probably because large parts of spoken language production are constituted by recurring syllables, e.g., in function words and bounded morphemes. As can be inferred from the Figure 1, the three patients with AOS showed a pattern that was comparable to that of the control persons.

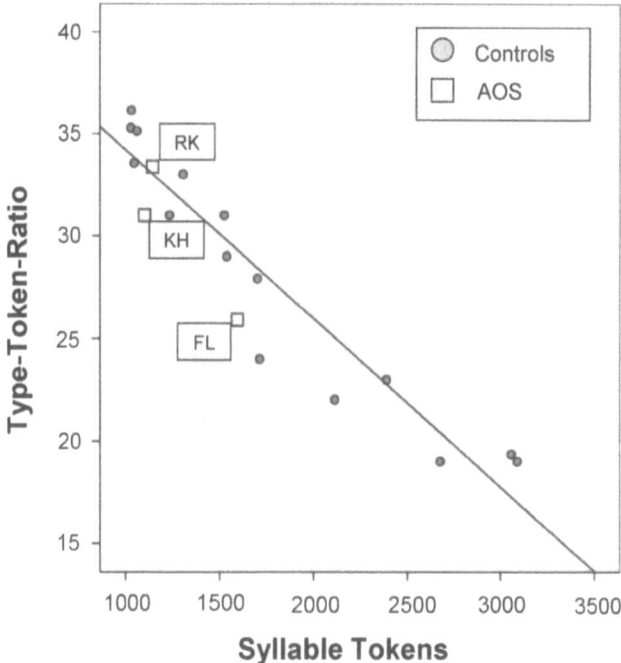

Figure 1. Type–Token ratio of canonical syllables, plotted against the number of syllable tokens for patients and healthy control participants. The solid line represents the linear regression function calculated for the normal participants (*N* = 15).

Distribution of syllable frequencies. For each participant the cumulative distribution of the frequency ranks of the target syllables was calculated from the "Database for Sublexical Frequencies and Structures", based on CELEX counts for spoken and written word forms (Aichert et al., 2007a). Syllable rank 1 corresponds to the most frequent syllable; the most infrequent syllable produced by a participant had rank 11047 (Figure 2). The solid horizontal line in Figure 2 marks the 85th percentile of the cumulative frequency distributions of all participants. The 85% criterion was chosen following Schiller (1997), who demonstrated that (in Dutch) approximately 85% of all syllable tokens in spoken language production can be covered by the 500 most frequent syllables. The small bar diagram included in Figure 2 shows that the participants included in our investigation reached the 85% threshold at similar rank values, i.e., between approximately 450 and 650. The three apraxic speakers fell within the normal range.

Distribution of syllable structures. Table 2 specifies the proportions of complex syllables, i.e., syllables in which at least one constituent (onset or coda) was a consonant cluster. Recall that canonical syllables were counted, hence these data do not reflect how the syllables were actually produced.

Two of the three apraxic speakers (RK, FL) produced a proportion of complex syllables comparable to that of the unimpaired controls. There was only one patient (KH) who used fewer complex syllables (15.6%) than did the normal participants.

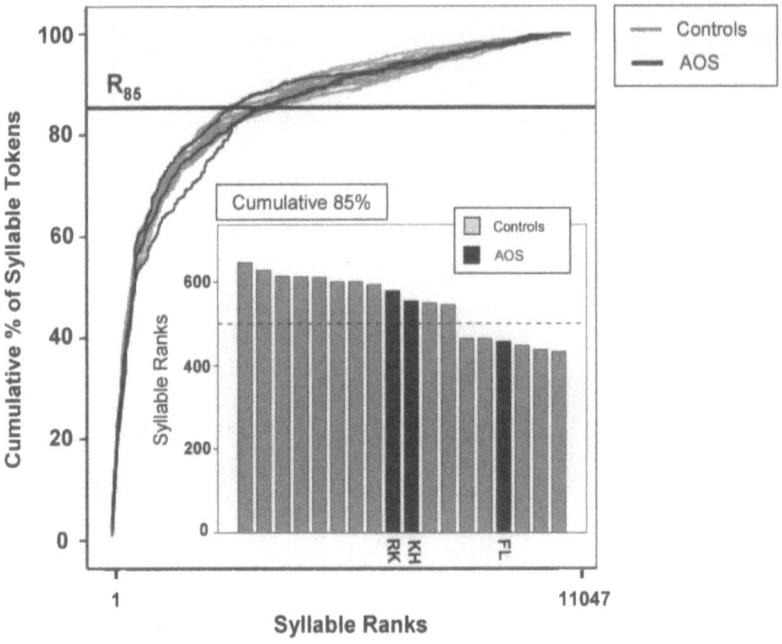

Figure 2. Cumulative frequencies of all (canonical) syllable tokens over syllable ranks for patients and healthy controls. The bar diagram insert plots the 85% thresholds of these distributions. The dashed line displays syllable rank 500.

TABLE 2
Absolute numbers and percentages of complex syllables

	Control persons (mean, range)	RK	FL	KH
N complex syllables	337 (169–610)	226	310	172
% complex syllables	18.8 (16.3–21.2)	19.7	19.4	15.6

Syllables containing at least one consonant cluster. For the control participants group mean values and ranges are specified.

Error analysis

Error analyses included only the patients' speech samples. The evaluation of errors was restricted to segmental errors and related to syllable units (thus quantity and position of errors within a syllable were neglected). The aim of the investigation was to reveal the influence of the factors syllable frequency and syllable complexity on the occurrence of errors in the apraxic speakers.

Influence of syllable frequency on error rates. In order to examine the influence of syllable frequency on the occurrence of errors, we first separated the set of canonical syllables into two frequency groups: syllables with ranks ≤ 250 (high-frequency) vs syllables with ranks > 250 (low-frequency). The threshold rank of 250 was chosen following the account by Aichert and Ziegler (2004). In the speech samples of the normal speakers examined here, the 250 most commonly used syllable types covered approximately 75% of the syllable tokens. Thus, these syllables were considered as being particularly overlearned. As can be inferred from Figure 3, all patients produced significantly more errors on low- than on high-frequency syllables (Pearson; RK: $\chi^2 = 28.3$; FL: $\chi^2 = 40.6$; KH: $\chi^2 = 10.5$; $p \leqslant .001$ in all cases).

Since high-frequency syllables tend to be less complex than low-frequency syllables, the data plotted in Figure 3 are contaminated by complexity effects. That is, in high-frequency syllables the proportion of complex syllables produced by the three apraxic patients was approximately 10% while in low-frequency syllables the proportion was approximately 40%. Therefore, the effect of syllable frequency was scrutinised anew on the basis of syllables with the same syllabic structure. We chose syllables with CVC structure, due to the fact that this structure appeared most frequently and, furthermore, was best balanced over the two frequency groups. The absolute numbers of CVC syllables depending on frequency groups as well as the absolute numbers/percentages of segmental errors are presented in Table 3.

In the CVC condition the error rates of all patients still indicated an advantage for high-frequency syllables. Therefore it can be concluded that there exists an influence of syllable frequency, which appears independent from syllable structure. A significant difference was found in two patients (Pearson; RK: $\chi^2 = 3.9$, $p < .05$; FL: $\chi^2 = 7.1$, $p < .01$). The advantage of high-frequency syllables failed to reach statistical significance in patient KH ($p > 0.5$).

Influence of syllable structure on error rates. To analyse the influence of syllable structure on the occurrence of segmental errors we first divided the canonical syllables of the speech samples into two categories: "complex" syllables, containing at least one consonant cluster (a complex onset, a complex coda, or both) and "simple" syllables, containing empty or non-branching onsets and codas. Figure 4 depicts the mean percentage of errors as a function of syllable structure. In all patients, a significant influence of complexity on accuracy was found (Pearson; RK: $\chi^2 = 8.5$, $p < .01$; FL: $\chi^2 = 10.8$, $p = .001$; KH: $\chi^2 = 8.4$, $p < .01$). This means, the patients seemed to benefit from simple syllable structures.

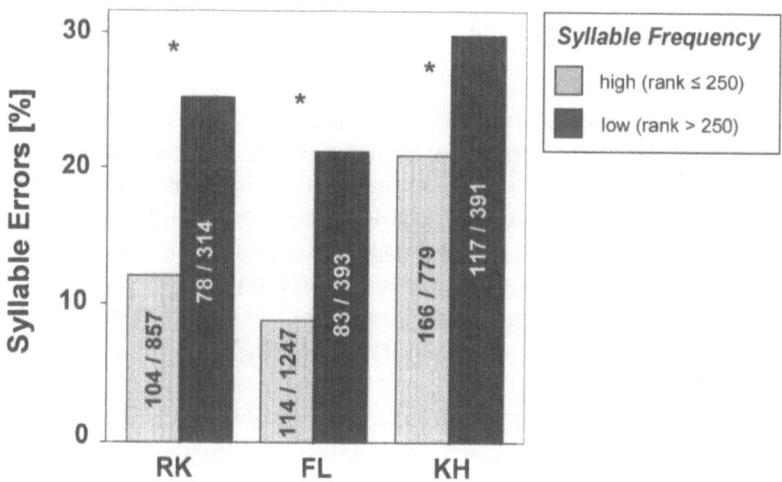

Figure 3. Proportion of errors on high-frequency syllables (syllable rank $\leqslant 250$) and low-frequency syllables (syllable rank > 250) per patient; the numbers printed in the bars specify absolute numbers of errors and syllables produced in each frequency class per patient.

TABLE 3
Influence of syllable frequency on apraxic errors (CVC syllables only)

Freq. group	RK		FL		KH	
	high	low	high	low	high	low
N_CVC	346	132	456	194	282	200
N_errors	50	29	44	33	71	57
% errors	14.5	22.0	9.6	17.0	25.2	28.5

N_CVC: number of syllable tokens with CVC structure per frequency group and patient; N_errors: number of errors occurring on syllables with CVC structure per frequency group and patient; % errors: percentage of errors occurring on syllables with CVC structure per frequency group and patient.

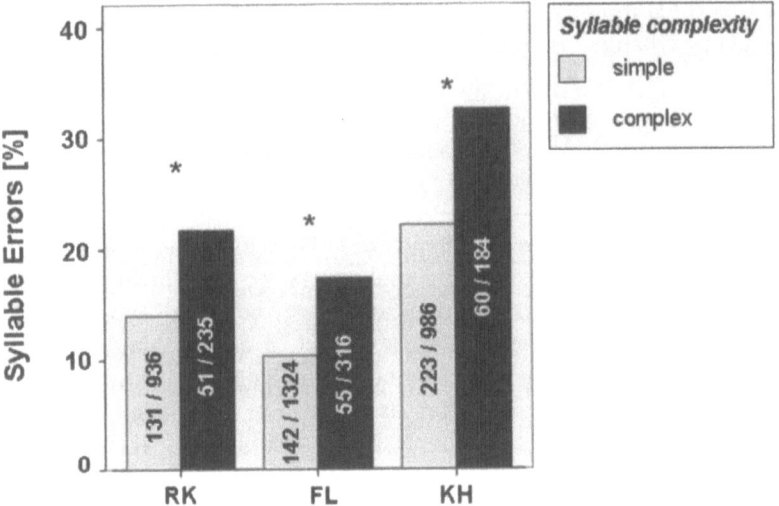

Figure 4. Influence of syllable complexity (simple vs complex) on error rates in RK, FL, and KH. The numbers printed in the bars specify the absolute numbers of errors and syllables produced in each complexity class per patient.

However, to compensate for the aforementioned interaction between syllable frequency and syllable structure, the complexity effect was re-examined separately for the categories of high- and low-frequency syllables (boundary rank 250; see above). In order to compare syllables with the same structural properties, we had to exclude low-frequency syllables whose degree of complexity did not occur among the high-frequency syllables. The excluded syllables contained either clusters with more than two phonemes (e.g., [ʃprʊŋ] Engl. "jump") or two clusters per syllable (e.g., [ʃprʊŋ] Engl. "jumps"). The numbers of excluded syllables were 26 for RK, 19 for FL, and 8 for KH.

Figure 5 represents the mean percentage of errors for each patient depending on syllable complexity and frequency. Within the low-frequency syllables (syllable rank > 250), the findings were as expected, with increased error rates on complex syllables in all patients. The effect reached statistical significance in FL and KH (Pearson; FL: $\chi^2 = 9.2$, $p < .01$; KH: $\chi^2 = 4.4$; $p < .05$) and showed a non-significant trend in RK ($\chi^2 = 3.5$; $p = .06$). However, no advantage of simple structures was

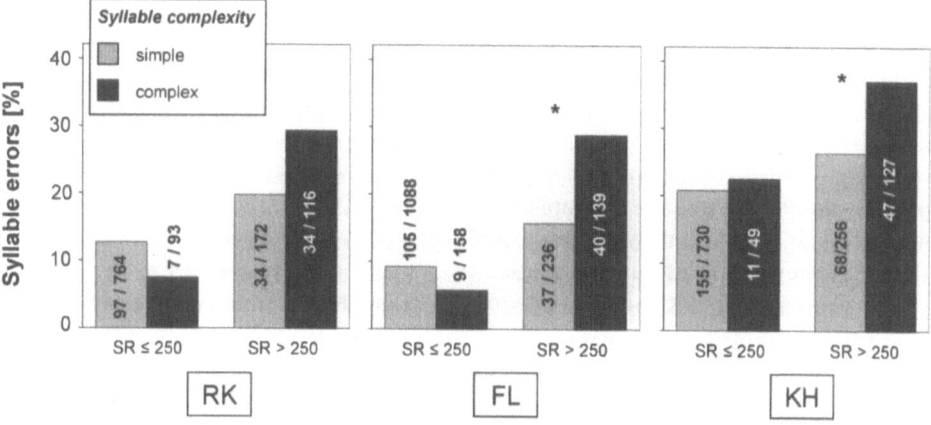

Figure 5. Influence of syllable complexity (simple vs complex) per patient. The figure shows mean errors rates in relation to high- (SR ⩽ 250) and low- (SR > 250) frequency syllables (SR: syllable rank); the numbers printed in the bars specify absolute numbers of errors and syllables per class (merged according to their frequency and complexity properties) and per patient.

found in the high-frequency syllables ($p > .05$ in all cases). Surprisingly, even a reduction of errors on the complex syllables (albeit not significant) was observed in two patients (RK, FL). It has to be added that the result persisted even after exclusion of very frequently occurring complex syllables, which are permitted to be reduced structurally by phonetic-phonological rule applications (e.g., [nɪçt] Engl. "not" > [nɪç]).

DISCUSSION

Previous studies investigating the influence of syllable frequency and syllable structure on the error rates in patients with AOS were almost exclusively based on single-word production tasks. As it is assumed that tasks like picture naming or word repetition differ substantially from natural speech production, our study addressed the influence of these sublexical parameters at the level of spontaneous speech. Since in spontaneous speech tasks patients deliberately select the speech units they produce, we first discuss the distribution properties of their speech samples, before we embark on their speech errors.

Distribution properties of the spontaneous speech samples

The Type–Token ratio, as a quantitative measure of the variation of syllable types in the speech samples, was similar in all participants, both the patients and the healthy controls. Regarding the distribution of the syllable frequencies the patients and the normal speakers showed comparable profiles, too. These findings are of particular importance since the normal variation in the selection of syllable types implied that the production of syllables was not restricted to a small number of frequently occurring syllable types. Furthermore, the data show that the patients did not circumvent low-frequency (hence, less overlearned) syllables.

Concerning the distribution of syllable structures, i.e., the proportion of structurally complex syllables, our results in patients RK and FL were consistent with those of the control persons. Although the complex units can be assumed to be "harder to articulate" and therefore more error prone, these patients did not evade producing them. By comparison, patient KH tended to produce fewer complex syllables than the healthy control persons. This finding might tentatively be interpreted as a strategy of bypassing motorically demanding syllables. In line with this assumption is an account by Edmonds and Marquardt (2004), who expected patients with AOS to have an implicit knowledge of their speech motor deficit that governs their selection of words, especially with respect to word length and syllable shape. However, finer-grained analyses of the structural properties in the apraxic patients revealed that KH in fact produced a reasonable number of complex onsets in her speech sample but her proportion of complex codas was clearly below average. At first sight this result may appear unexpected, since commonly the onset position has been considered especially challenging for patients with AOS (e.g., Aichert & Ziegler, 2004; Canter et al., 1985). As mentioned earlier, patient KH had a concomitant residual aphasic impairment, which was manifest mainly in a mild agrammatism. Thus it cannot be ruled out that the low rate of complex codas was actually due to a partial avoidance of utterances requiring grammatical *flexion*, which, in German, often results in complex word endings.

Error analysis

Influence of syllable frequency. One of the major results of this study was that the error susceptibility in the spontaneous speech production of patients with AOS was influenced by syllable frequency. In each of the patients examined here, the proportion of errors produced over all syllable structures was significantly higher on low- than on high-frequency syllables. That is, syllables that, due to their high frequency of occurrence, are considered particularly overlearned, were produced more accurately by the participants. In two patients (RK, FL) this effect even remained stable when we confined our analysis to syllables with CVC sequences, thereby ruling out any confound with syllable structure. However, in patient KH the significant effect of syllable frequency disappeared in the CVC condition, which points to the strong interaction between these two sublexical parameters. Nevertheless, this patient too showed an advantage in the production of high-frequency syllables.

This result is a replication of the findings reported by Aichert and Ziegler (2004) who were the first to describe a syllable frequency effect in AOS speakers. The data reported here are remarkable for the fact that they applied to carefully selected AOS patients on a single-case basis, while Aichert and Ziegler (2004) reported group statistics. Moreover, they relate to spontaneous speech rather than word repetition, which renders them particularly valid. This provides strong evidence for the assumptions mentioned earlier, namely that patients with AOS do use a syllabic encoding mechanism, which—according to Levelt's model—includes access to the precompiled gestural scores in a mental syllabary. Otherwise, no influence of syllable-related parameters on accuracy would have been found. As a consequence, the occurrence of errors must be explained by an at least partial damage of the articulatory-phonetic programmes stored in the syllabary. Even though we have no positive evidence concerning the nature of this damage, one might speculate that the motor specifications in these programs are incomplete or distorted. Such a pathomechanism would be compatible with symptoms like articulatory groping, phonetic distortions, or close-to-target substitutions. Irrespective of this interpretation, however, our data underpin the notion of a frequency-based hierarchical organisation of the mental syllabary, since high-frequency syllables were relatively better preserved than low-frequency syllables.

As mentioned above, one of the three patients with AOS (KH) only showed a minor influence of syllable frequency when syllable structure was controlled for. How can this result be interpreted? One may speculate that KH's results were more strongly influenced by contextual factors since she produced a substantial number of contextually driven errors, mainly anticipations, in her spontaneous speech.[1] Although we are not yet able to answer the question of why contextual factors should affect some speakers more than others, it will certainly be worthwhile to pay more attention to between-word phenomena in the future, since the occurrence of environmental errors might possibly attenuate the effect of syllable frequency, considering that this error type concerns high- and low-frequency syllables alike.

Influence of syllable structure. Over and above the effect of syllable frequency, we found a strong influence of syllable structure on error rates in the spontaneous speech of all participating patients. It can be inferred from this result that syllables that comprise intra-syllabic clusters are articulatorily demanding and therefore have an impact on production accuracy. This finding too is comparable with the results of single word studies (e.g., Romani & Galluzzi, 2005). However, a detailed analysis, conducted to disentangle the confounding parameters syllable structure and syllable frequency, revealed a more differentiated pattern, since no influence of syllable structure was found among the high-frequency syllables.

The opposite (and actually the expected) pattern was found among the low-frequency syllables. Here, the complexity of syllables had an apparent impact on error rates, resulting in a higher vulnerability of the complex units. We infer from these observations that high-frequency syllables may be overlearned to such an extent that an increasing degree of complexity will not affect their production. The opposite seems to be true for syllables with lower frequencies of occurrence, since they possess lower degrees of overlearnedness.

However, these findings are not easily accounted for by Levelt's postulate of a mental syllabary comprising holistically stored motor patterns, since effects of syllable structure have not been addressed in this model. In accordance with the conclusions drawn by Romani and Galluzzi (2005) our results support the assumption that the syllabary holds an internal organisation with respect to syllable complexity. More concretely, we may interpret the motor patterns stored in the syllabary as arranged along a continuum, with structurally simple, high-frequency syllables constituting the most accessible and least vulnerable ones and structurally complex, low-frequency syllables being particularly unstable (see also Aichert & Ziegler, 2008 this issue).

---

[1] Some authors ascribed these errors to a concomitant aphasic-phonological impairment (e.g., Itoh & Sasanuma, 1984; McNeill, Pratt, & Fossett, 2004), but the observation of anticipatory as well as of perseveratory and transposition errors also coincides with many common descriptions of AOS (e.g., Dabul, 2000; Darley et al., 1975; La Pointe & Johns, 1975; Wertz, La Pointe, & Rosenbek, 1984).

CONCLUSION

We found that articulatory accuracy in the spontaneous speech production of patients with AOS was influenced by the same factors as in single-word tasks, i.e., syllable frequency and syllable structure. From our results the following conclusions can be drawn: The factors syllable frequency and syllable structure are consistently influential, even across different modalities of speech production. Therefore, approaches based on single-word processing tasks are to a certain extent capable of detecting the factors that also influence conversational speech. However, this conclusion has to be amended by the fact that natural, spontaneous speech production involves motor planning processes operating across words. The data presented here provide first indications that the error patterns of at least some speakers with AOS may disclose dysfunction at this processing level. This makes investigations of phrase-level or conversational speech an important avenue to follow in future studies of AOS.

REFERENCES

Aichert, I., Marquardt, C., & Ziegler, W. (2005). Frequenzen sublexikalischer einheiten des Deutschen: CELEX-basierte Datenbanken. *Neurolinguistik, 19*, 5–31.

Aichert, I., Marquardt, C., & Ziegler, W. (unpublished). Computer program for the construction and analysis of speech material. EKN, München: EKN.

Aichert, I., & Ziegler, W. (2004). Syllable frequency and syllable structure in apraxia of speech. *Brain and Language, 88*, 148–159.

Aichert, I., & Ziegler, W. (2008). Learning a syllable from its parts: Cross-syllabic generalisation effects in patients with apraxia of speech. *Aphasiology, 22*, 1216–1229.

Baayen, R. H., Piepenbrock, R., & Gulikers, L. (1995). *The CELEX lexical database* [CD-ROM]. Philadelphia: Linguistic Data Consortium, University of Pennsylvania.

Canter, G. J., Trost, J. E., & Burns, M. S. (1985). Contrasting speech patterns in apraxia of speech and phonemic paraphasia. *Brain and Language, 24*, 204–222.

Carreiras, M., & Perea, M. (2004). Naming pseudowords in Spanish: Effects of syllable frequency. *Brain and Language, 90*, 393–400.

Cholin, J. (2008). The mental syllabary in speech production: An integration of different approaches and domains. *Aphasiology, 22*, 1127–1141.

Cholin, J., Levelt, W. J. M., & Schiller, N. O. (2006). Effects of syllable frequency in speech production. *Cognition, 99*, 205–235.

Clements, G. N., & Keyser, S. J. (1983). *CV phonology: A generative theory of the syllable*. Cambridge, MA: MIT Press.

Code, C. (1998). Major review: Models, theories and heuristics in apraxia of speech. *Clinical Linguistics and Phonetics, 12*, 47–65.

Dabul, B. L. (2000). *Apraxia Battery for Adults – Second edition (ABA-2)*. Austin, TX: Pro-ED, Inc.

Darley, F. L., Aronson, A. E., & Brown, J. R. (1975). *Motor speech disorders*. Philadelphia: W. B. Saunders.

Edmonds, L. A., & Marquardt, T. P. (2004). Syllable use in apraxia of speech: Preliminary findings. *Aphasiology, 18*, 1121–1134.

Huber, W., Poeck, K., Weniger, D., & Willmes, K. (1983). *Aachener Aphasie Test (AAT)*. Göttingen: Hogrefe.

Itoh, M., & Sasanuma, S. (1984). Articulatory movements in apraxia of speech. In J. C. Rosenbek, M. R. McNeil, & A. E. Aronson (Eds.), *Apraxia of speech: Physiology, acoustics, linguistics, management* (pp. 135–165). San Diego: College-Hill Press.

Kohler, K. J. (1990). Segmental reduction in connected speech in German: Phonological facts and phonetic explanations. In W. J. Hardcastle & A. Marchal (Eds.), *Speech production and speech modelling* (pp. 69–92). Dordrecht: Kluwer.

Kohler, K. J. (2001). The investigation of connected speech processes. Theory, method, hypotheses and empirical data. In K. J. Kohler (Ed.), *AIPUK 35. Sound patterns in German read and spontaneous speech: Symbolic structures and gestural dynamics* (pp. 1–32). Kiel: IPDS.

Kohn, S. E., & Smith, K. L. (1990). Between-word speech errors in conduction aphasia. *Cognitive Neuropsychology, 7*, 133–156.

La Pointe, L. L., & Johns, D. F. (1975). Some phonemic characteristics in apraxia of speech. *Journal of Communication Disorders, 8*, 259–269.

Laganaro, M. (2005). Syllable frequency effect in speech production: Evidence from aphasia. *Journal of Neurolinguistics, 18*, 221–235.

Laganaro, M. (2008). Is there a syllable frequency effect in aphasia or in apraxia of speech or both? *Aphasiology, 22*, 1191–1200.

Laganaro, M., & Alario, F. X. (2006). On the locus of the syllable frequency effect in speech production. *Journal of Memory and Language, 55*, 178–196.

Levelt, W. J. M., Roelofs, A., & Meyer, A. S. (1999). A theory of lexical access in speech production. *Behavioral and Brain Sciences, 22*, 1–75.

Levelt, W. J. M., & Wheeldon, L. R. (1994). Do speakers have access to a mental syllabary? *Cognition, 50*, 239–269.

Liepold, M., Ziegler, W., & Brendel, B. (2003). *Hierarchische Wortlisten. Ein Nachsprechtest für die Sprechapraxiediagnostik*. Dortmund: Borgmann.

McNeil, M. R., Pratt, S. R., & Fossett, T. R. D. (2004). The differential diagnosis of apraxia of speech. In B. Maassen, R. D. Kent, H. F. M. Peters, P. H. van Lieshout, & W. Hulstijn (Eds.), *Speech motor control in normal and disordered speech* (pp. 389–413). Oxford, UK: Oxford University Press.

Nespoulous, J-L., Joanette, Y., Beland, R., Caplan, D., & Lecours, A. R. (1984). Phonological disturbances in aphasia: Is there a "markedness effect" in aphasic phonemic errors? In F. C. Rose (Ed.), *Advances in aphasiology, Vol. 42: Progress in aphasiology* (pp. 203–214). London: Raven Press.

Nickels, L., & Howard, D. (2000). When the words won't come: Relating impairments and models of spoken word production. In L. Wheeldon (Ed.), *Aspects of language production* (pp. 115–142). Hove, UK: Psychology Press.

Nickels, L., & Howard, D. (2004). Dissociating effects of number of phonemes, number of syllables, and syllabic complexity on word production in aphasia: It's the number of phonemes that counts. *Cognitive Neuropsychology, 21*, 57–78.

Odell, K., McNeil, M., Rosenbek, J. C., & Hunter, L. (1990). Perceptual characteristics of consonant production by apraxic speakers. *Journal of Speech and Hearing Disorders, 55*, 345–359.

Romani, C., & Calabrese, A. (1998). Syllabic constraints in the phonological errors of an aphasic patient. *Brain and Language, 64*, 83–121.

Romani, C., & Galluzzi, C. (2005). Effects of syllabic complexity in predicting accuracy of repetition and direction of errors in patients with articulatory and phonological difficulties. *Cognitive Neuropsychology, 22*, 817–850.

Rosenbek, J. C., Kent, R. D., & La Pointe, L. L. (1984). Apraxia of speech: An overview and some perspectives. In J. C. Rosenbek, M. R. McNeil, & A. E. Aronson (Eds.), *Apraxia of speech: Physiology, acoustics, linguistics, management* (pp. 1–72). San Diego: College-Hill Press.

Schiller, N. O. (1997). *The role of the syllable in speech production. MPI Series in Psycholinguistics.* Nijmegen: MPI for Psycholinguistik.

Shattuck-Hufnagel, S. (1992). The role of word structure in segmental serial ordering. *Cognition, 42*, 213–259.

Stemberger, J. P. (1990). Wordshape errors in language production. *Cognition, 35*, 123–157.

Stemberger, J. P. (1991). Apparent anti-frequency effects in language production: The addition bias and phonological underspecification. *Journal of Memory and Language, 30*, 161–185.

Stemberger, J. P., & Treiman, R. (1986). The internal structure of word-initial consonant clusters. *Journal of Memory and Language, 25*, 163–180.

Trost, J. E., & Canter, G. J. (1974). Apraxia of speech in patients with Broca's sphasia: A study of phoneme production accuracy and error patterns. *Brain and Language, 1*, 63–79.

Varley, R., & Whiteside, S. P. (2001). What is the underlying impairment in acquired apraxia of speech? *Aphasiology, 15*, 39–49.

Wertz, R. T., La Pointe, L. L., & Rosenbek, J. C. (1984). *Apraxia of speech in adults: The disorder and its management*. Orlando, FL: Grune & Stratton.

Ziegler, W. (2002). Psycholinguistic and motor theories of apraxia of speech. *Seminars in Speech and Language, 23*, 231–243.

APHASIOLOGY, 2008, 22 (11), 1216–1229

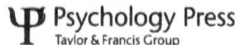

Learning a syllable from its parts: Cross-syllabic generalisation effects in patients with apraxia of speech

Ingrid Aichert and Wolfram Ziegler

City Hospital Bogenhausen, München, Germany

Background: The impairment underlying apraxia of speech (AOS) is usually attributed to the phonetic encoding stage of the speech production process, where speech motor programs are accessed (e.g., Code, 1998). At this processing stage, Levelt, Roelofs, and Meyer (1999) postulate a store of motor patterns for frequently used syllables ("syllabary"). These syllable gestures are assumed to be holistically represented. However, the fact that syllable structure influences the error mechanism of AOS is in conflict with the assumption of holistic syllable gestures.

Aims: This study examined the assumption of *holistic* syllable-sized motor programs in apraxia of speech by a learning paradigm. We investigated if training of phonologically simple syllables, which were derived from more complex target syllables, showed a generalisation effect on these target syllables. If the assumption of holistic syllable programs is appropriate, no generalisation effects are expected.

Methods & Procedures: A learning experiment was conducted with four patients with AOS. For each of 24 complex target syllables a set of 15 training syllables was derived by deleting one or two of the onset and/or coda consonants or by assimilating consonantal features. The learning trials comprised repetitions of the training syllables, block-wise for each target syllable. To assess generalisation effects, segmental errors and disfluencies were counted and syllable durations were measured before and immediately after training, for the target syllables as well as for matched control syllables.

Outcomes & Results: In the patients as a group, the training resulted in significant and specific improvements on the complex target syllables. The strongest effect was found in RK, a patient with pure AOS. This patient additionally exhibited a significant reduction of target but not of control syllable durations.

Conclusions: In this learning study, patients with apraxia of speech showed specific generalisation effects from phonologically simple syllables to more complex syllables. These effects cannot be explained by the assumption of holistically stored syllable programs (Levelt et al., 1999). In contrast, the results suggest that syllabic motor programs comprise an internal phonological structure.

Keywords: Apraxia of speech; Syllable; Motor learning; Generalisation.

Address correspondence to: Ingrid Aichert, EKN – Clinical Neuropsychology Research Group, Dachauer Str. 164, 80992 München, Germany. E-mail: ingrid.aichert@extern.lrz-muenchen.de

The first author of this study was supported by a grant from the German research foundation (Zi 469/6–2). We are grateful to the patients for their participation. We would also like to thank the speech therapists from the following clinical institutions for their participation and collaboration on clinical issues: Neuropsychological Department/City Hospital München-Bogenhausen, Neurological Clinic Bad Aibling, Rehabilitation Hospital Lenggries, Speech Pathology Practice Seith/München. ReHa-Hilfe e.V. is acknowledged for continuing support.

Apraxia of speech (AOS) is defined as a disorder of speech motor programming. It is characterised by phonemic and phonetic errors, articulatory groping, difficulties in initiating speech, and prosodic abnormalities (see Code, 1998; Croot, 2002; McNeil, Robin, & Schmidt, 1997). Despite an increased understanding of the speech motor system in current models of speech production, the pathomechanism underlying AOS is still under discussion (e.g., Miller, 2000; Ziegler, 2002). One specific question concerns the size of speech motor programs that are accessible to patients with AOS.

Modern discussions of AOS have related the apraxic impairment to the phonetic encoding stage of the speech production process, as modelled by Levelt, Roelofs, and Meyer (1999) (e.g., Nickels & Howard, 2000; Ziegler, 2002, 2007). The linguistic unit that is at the core of speech motor programming in Levelt's model is the *syllable*. It is postulated that during phonetic encoding speakers access a long-term store of "gestural scores" for the frequently occurring syllables of their language; i.e., they download the motor information for each syllable as a pre-compiled, holistic package. Infrequent or new syllables have no holistically stored phonetic code and must therefore be assembled on-line from smaller, sub-syllabic units ("segment-by-segment assembly", Levelt et al., 1999, p. 32). Evidence for such a store of ready-made syllable programs comes from psycholinguistic studies, in which normal participants produced high-frequent syllables with shorter response latencies than low-frequent syllables (Cholin, Levelt, & Schiller, 2006; Levelt & Wheeldon, 1994). The assumption of the mental syllabary is strengthened by other theories, which view the syllable as a basic speech unit (e.g., Crompton, 1982; Lindblom, 1983) and by the fact that syllables have been considered as the first units of motor control in speech acquisition (e.g., MacNeilage, Davis, Kinney, & Matyear, 2000). Hence, with regard to apraxia of speech the question arises whether these patients are still using syllabic units for speech motor programming.

We recently demonstrated an influence of syllable frequency on the error production of patients with AOS, who proved to be more accurate on frequent syllables than on infrequent ones. Moreover, we found that the occurrence of a certain error type in these patients, i.e., cluster reduction, was heavily dependent on the position of the cluster within a word (Aichert & Ziegler, 2004). Specifically, two clusters separated by a syllable boundary were reduced less often than intra-syllabic clusters. The fact that apraxic speakers were influenced by syllabic factors led to the conclusion that patients with AOS still have access to the mental syllabary, but that the syllabic programs must be partly destroyed. The degree to which stored movement information is available to them depends on syllable frequency and syllable structure. However, this conclusion is at odds with Levelt's model, which postulates that the entries in the mental syllabary are holistic units, i.e., "complete gestural programs" (Levelt et al., 1999, p. 32). In this theory, the internal structure of syllables is not considered relevant at the phonetic encoding stage, since in Levelt and Wheeldon's (1994) study naming latencies in normal speakers were influenced by syllable frequency, but not by syllable complexity.

That syllable structure counts in patients with AOS has been reported many times. Apraxic patients are known to produce higher error rates on syllables containing consonant clusters as compared to syllables containing only single consonants (e.g., Canter, Trost, & Burns, 1985; Odell, McNeil, Rosenbek, & Hunter, 1990; Romani & Galluzzi, 2005), and to simplify complex syllable structures by deleting consonants in clusters (e.g., Aichert & Ziegler, 2004; Canter et al., 1985; Odell et al., 1990; Romani & Galluzzi, 2005; Staiger & Ziegler, 2008 this issue). Hence, if apraxic patients are sensitive to the syllabic architecture of words and if, at the same time, the complexity of a syllable influences their articulatory accuracy, the assumption of holistic syllable plans cannot be upheld. Therefore, Romani and Galluzzi (2005, p. 845) concluded that "the syllable units in the syllabary should be organized according to complexity so that simple syllables are easier to access than more complex syllables".

In the study reported here we embarked on the question of holistic programs for syllables from a new perspective, i.e., with a learning paradigm. In this approach, we exploited the fact that apraxic patients make many errors on complex syllables and may therefore be trained to improve their accuracy on such items. More specifically, we investigated if the learning of a complex syllable can be based on training of smaller and simpler fractions of it.

Using this approach we pursued a twofold aim: First, we continued earlier attempts at revealing the units on which the apraxic speech mechanism operates, and at describing the structural make-up of these units (cf. Ziegler, 2005). Second, we addressed an important issue of the treatment research that has been undertaken in this field so far—the issue of the most appropriate treatment units. In theory-based treatment approaches for apraxia of speech, the discussion about units to be chosen as treatment targets should be guided by hypotheses about the programming units impaired in AOS (cf. Odell, 2002). Previous treatment studies have selected target units of very different sizes, i.e., single segments (e.g., Dabul & Bollier, 1976), syllables, multisyllabic words, or short phrases (e.g., Bose, Square, Schlosser, & van Lieshout, 2001; Brendel & Ziegler, 2008; Freed, Marshall, & Frazier, 1997).

Current knowledge about the pathomechanism of AOS, as outlined above, strongly suggests that syllables are good candidates as treatment targets in the remediation of apraxia of speech. If, as the theory of Levelt et al. (1999) postulates, phonetic syllables must be considered as *holistically* stored motor patterns, treatments based on syllable-sized units would be efficient only for syllables that are actually exercised during therapy (training effect), whereas *generalisation effects* from trained syllables to structurally related, but untrained, syllables cannot be expected. In practice, this would imply that every single syllable of the syllabary needs to be trained separately with a patient.

In the present study we investigated if this is indeed the case. We selected a set of complex target syllables to be learned by apraxic patients and devised, for each of them, a set of structurally less complex derivatives that were used for training. Our question was whether the untrained root syllable benefits from training of its descendants. As an example, we asked if a patient's articulation of a complex syllable like [trant] improves when she/he exercises syllables like [ran], [rant], [tran] etc. If this occurs—i.e., syllables can be learned from their parts—we can infer that syllabic motor programs are not primitives. So far, the ongoing learning experiment has been conducted with four apraxic speakers, one of them showing a pure form of AOS.

METHOD

Participants

Four patients with AOS[1] were examined. All participants were right-handed native speakers of German who had suffered infarctions in the region of the left middle

---

[1] Two patients, RK and KH, also participated in an investigation of spontaneous speech by Staiger & Ziegler (2008 this issue). However, the two studies were undertaken at two different points in time.

cerebral artery. All patients were in a post-acute or chronic stage between 2 and 41 months post-onset. The diagnosis of AOS was based on the following criteria: occurrence of phonemic errors (sound substitutions, anticipations, and perseverations), phonetic distortions, articulatory groping, difficulties in initiating speech due to false starts and restarts, and prosodic deviations such as overall slow speech rate and intersyllabic pauses (McNeil et al., 1997).

Two patients, RK and KH, demonstrated mild-to-moderate AOS with virtually no aphasia as revealed by the Aachener Aphasie Test, a standardised German aphasia test (AAT; Huber, Poeck, Weniger, & Willmes, 1983). The other two participants, LF and MK, were moderately disturbed regarding speech apraxic symptoms. Both patients were classified as having a concomitant mild-to-moderate Broca's aphasia. In three patients no signs of dysarthria were evident; only LF exhibited a residual dysarthric impairment.

All diagnoses were made by experienced speech and language therapists. They were confirmed by the diagnostic assessments conducted in the context of the present study. Table 1 outlines the patients' data.

RK was diagnosed as having a pure, mild-to-moderate AOS with no aphasic impairment. The AAT (Huber et al., 1983) was entirely unremarkable and there were no indications of syntactic, lexical, or morphological impairments in speech production or of impaired comprehension. His speech-apraxic symptoms were evident in all speech production tasks. Spontaneous speech, repetition, naming, and reading aloud were characterised by numerous segmental errors, i.e., phonemic errors and phonetic distortions, which occurred inconsistently. Concerning the suprasegmental level, RK showed a slow speech rate due to syllable segregation in multisyllabic words, lengthened segments, and intrusive schwa productions in words with complex syllable structures. Moreover, articulatory groping and self-corrections also contributed to an overall reduced speech rate. The impression of a remarkably effortful speech was caused, among other factors, by an exertion of the facial muscles, increased loudness, and by RK's frequent attempts to self-correct his speech errors. Generally, RK seemed to continuously take pains to avoid segmental errors, resulting in a controlled manner of speaking.

TABLE 1
Clinical data

	RK	KH	LF	MK
Age	49	65	59	49
Gender	m	f	m	m
Months post-onset	4	2	7	41
AOS: Severity score[a]	mild-to-moderate	mild-to-moderate	moderate	moderate
Aphasia classification	no aphasia[b]	no aphasia[b, c]	Broca's aphasia[d] (mild-to-moderate)	Broca's aphasia[d] (mild-to-moderate)

[a]According to clinical judgement.   [b]Classification based on AAT (Aachener Aphasie Test) screening, which aims to differentiate between patients with and without aphasia (Huber et al., 1983). [c]Analysis of spontaneous speech and a clinical test examining text comprehension revealed residual aphasic deficits.   [d]Classification based on AAT (Huber et al., 1983).

Patient KH exhibited a mild-to-moderate AOS and, according to the AAT (Huber et al., 1983), no concomitant aphasia. Yet residual aphasic impairments, undetected by the AAT, became evident in spontaneous speech. In particular, signs of agrammatism and few word-finding difficulties were observed. Furthermore, written text comprehension was mildly disturbed. AOS was predominantly diagnosed on the basis of numerous phonemic errors and phonetic distortions. KH's speech exhibited a rather normal prosodic structure at the word level, with only few intersyllabic pauses and sound prolongations. However, her overall oral fluency was affected due to articulatory groping and frequent self-corrections.

Patient LF demonstrated a moderate AOS with a concomitant Broca's aphasia (AAT, Huber et al., 1983) and with residual signs of dysarthria. His comprehension abilities were mildly disturbed as evidenced in text-level tasks. In spontaneous speech he used mostly two- to three-word sentences. This, pattern was not interpreted as agrammatic by nature, since LF was grammatically almost undisturbed in reading aloud. Rather, his reduced syntax in spontaneous speech was interpreted as an adaptation to his articulatory problems. Relating to his dysarthria, reduced articulatory strength, especially of stop consonants, could be observed. However, in isolation he was able to produce all consonants correctly. Overall, his speech impairment was dominated by apraxic signs: he produced many segmental errors, and syllables with a complex consonant structure were frequently simplified by elisions. Numerous self-corrections as well as visible groping and other forms of initiation difficulties led to a breakdown of overall speech fluency.

MK was diagnosed as having moderate AOS and a mild-to-moderate Broca's aphasia (AAT, Huber et al., 1983). Minor comprehension deficits could be observed at the sentence and the text level. He experienced word-finding difficulties, which were particularly apparent in spontaneous speech. Regarding syntactic structure, the patient frequently produced short and simple sentences. However, his expressive abilities were dominated by his apraxic errors: The spontaneous speech of MK was mainly characterised by segmental errors, which nearly exclusively occurred at word onset. Clusters were frequently reduced. Groping behaviour was rare, which may be attributed to the patient's long-term adaptation to his disorder (more than 3 years). On occasion he attempted to self-correct, and in longer words a scanning speech rhythm could be observed.

Since the experiment reported here was based on a word-repetition task, deficits in auditory perception had to be excluded. An auditory discrimination test with non-words from the LeMo battery (De Bleser, Cholewa, Stadie, & Tabatabaie, 2004) revealed intact auditory processing abilities in all patients (RK: 71/72 correct; KH: 66/72 correct; LF: 72/72 correct; MK: 72/72 correct).

Materials

Target syllables. The target syllables consisted of 24 common monosyllabic nouns and verbs with a complex syllable structure. Each item comprised a consonant cluster in syllable onset and coda position with two or three consonants per cluster (for examples see Table 2).

The item list was controlled for word and syllable frequency. Whereas word frequency counts were directly taken from the German corpus of the CELEX database (Baayen, Piepenbrock, & Gulikers, 1995), syllable frequencies had to be

TABLE 2
Monosyllabic target items with complex syllable structure ($N = 24$)

Syllable structure	Examples
CCVCC ($N = 16$)	knast (jail)
	pʁaχt (pomp)
	ʃlɛ:ft ((he) sleeps)
CCCVCC/CCVCCC ($N = 8$)	tʁɪŋst ((you) drink)
	ʃtaunst ((you) marvel)
	ʃtʁaut(beach)

calculated on the basis of these word frequencies (Aichert, Marquardt, & Ziegler, unpublished database 2007).[2] All but four target words were low-frequent, and all syllables were ranked as low frequent as well.[3]

Training syllables. For each target syllable a set of 15 training syllables was derived by deleting one or two of the onset and/or coda consonants, thereby reducing the onset and/or coda clusters of the target syllables to single consonants. As an example, among the training syllables for the target word /knast/ (engl. *jail*) were the syllables /kas/, /nat/, /nast/ or /knat/. Empty positions resulting from omissions of complete clusters were avoided. In some of the training items the onset or coda cluster was further simplified by assimilating place or manner of articulation of adjacent consonants. For example, two training items for the target syllable /knast/ used the onset /kl/, assimilating the second consonant for the feature "oral". The simplifications of the target syllables frequently, but not always, resulted in neologisms.

Procedure

The 24 target items were trained within two sessions. Half of the items served as target items in the first session, the other half was used as control items. Control items and target items were interchanged in the second session. As a result of this procedure, every item served as both a target syllable and a control syllable. Since only immediate effects were assessed, effects of the order of item presentation could be neglected (see below).

Training. For each target syllable, the derived training syllables were presented block-wise. In total, 12 learning blocks were conducted in each session, one for each target syllable. Within a learning block, the patient successively repeated the training syllables after oral presentation by the examiner (the first author). The training items were ordered from phonologically most simple (e.g., /kas/) to most complex (e.g., /knat/). In case of an error on one of the training syllables, various therapeutic techniques were used to facilitate the correct articulatory pattern (e.g.,

[2] This German syllable frequency database comprises 11060 syllable entries, with /di:/ as the most frequent syllable in German assigned with frequency rank 1.
[3] Range of word frequency (frequency per mio.): 0-81 (median = 1). Range of syllable frequency (ranks): 654–10961 (median = 4542). For arguments regarding the classification of syllables as low frequency and high frequency, respectively, see Staiger and Ziegler (2008 this issue).

articulatory placement, integral stimulation). The examiner also provided feedback regarding suprasegmental failures (intersegmental pauses or phoneme lengthenings) by encouraging the patients to speak faster or more fluently. Each training syllable could be repeated up to three times before the next syllable was presented for repetition. The full target forms never occurred during the training sessions.

Assessment of immediate generalisation effects. To assess generalisation effects, the target syllable and a control syllable of comparable complexity were presented for repetition immediately before and after each learning block. Over both sessions, a total of 24 target syllables and 24 control syllables were examined.

Data analysis

The patients' responses were recorded on video or audiotape (microphone: Beyerdynamic TG-X-58, video camera: Panasonic NV-GS180, digital voice recorder: Sanyo *ICR-B175NX*) and were later auditorily evaluated by the first author. The target and control syllables produced immediately before and after a learning block were transcribed using broad phonetic transcription. Additionally, acoustic measures of syllable duration were obtained using wideband spectograms (Praat 4.2).

For evaluation, each syllable was first analysed with respect to correct/incorrect production, independent of error quality. In a second, finer-grained analysis, errors were classified as segmental and suprasegmental, respectively. Segmental errors included phonetic distortions, substitutions, additions, omissions, or combinations thereof. Suprasegmental errors comprised phoneme lengthenings and intersegmental pauses. We considered whole syllables as error units, i.e., multiple deviations on one syllable were counted as a single error.

Acoustic syllable durations were measured by determining the onset of the initial and the offset of the final phoneme. Items whose syllable structure was altered (i.e., by elisions or additions of onset or coda consonants, respectively) were not included in the syllable duration measurements. To be able to compare the syllable durations produced by the patients with those produced by normal speakers we additionally examined six controls (three male, three female; age, mean: 46.3, range: 30–54) who repeated each target syllable twice, resulting in a total of 48 probes for each participant (total: $N = 288$).

In order to assess the reliability of the auditory and acoustic analyses, 20% of the target syllables from each participants were re-analysed (total: $N = 240$). Equal proportions were selected from the probes produced before and after the learning trials, respectively. A second, experienced listener first transcribed the items to assess the perceptually based error categories and afterwards conducted the duration measurements for these items. There was a significant agreement between the two transcribers for the overall error rate ($\kappa = .89$, $p < .001$) and for the segmental errors ($\kappa = .90$, $p < .001$). However, there was a greater discrepancy in the ratings for the suprasegmental errors, even though these judgements were still contingent to a statistically significant extent ($\kappa = .51$, $p < .001$). Regarding syllable duration analyses, a high correlation between the values measured by the two examiners was found (Pearson Correlation, $r = .977$, $p < .001$).

RESULTS

Perceived errors

Before training, there was no significant difference between overall error numbers on the syllables serving as targets and controls, respectively (target: 52%, control: 43%; $\chi^2 = 1.69$, $p > .05$).[4] Overall, most errors were produced on the onset clusters (onset errors: 66%, nucleus errors: 6%, coda errors: 28%). In both onset and coda position, substitution errors were prevalent (onset substitutions: 69%; coda substitutions: 62%), but the patients also produced a relatively high proportion of elisions (31% vs 38%).

Regarding training effects, overall error rates for the target syllables decreased significantly from 52% before to 27% after the learning trials (McNemar, one-sided; $\chi^2 = 15.56$, $p < .001$). For the control syllables, on the contrary, there was even an increased error rate (43% before vs 57% after learning; $\chi^2 = 8.76$, $p < .01$). After the training sessions, error proportions on the two item groups differed significantly (targets: 27%, controls: 57%; $\chi^2 = 17.96$, $p < .001$).

When the target syllables were analysed separately for segmental and suprasegmental errors, a significant effect was only obtained for the segmental errors (43% before vs 23% after training; $\chi^2 = 10.62$, $p < .001$). Suprasegmental errors decreased as well (from 10% before to 4% after training), but absolute numbers were too small for statistical testing. For the control syllables, the rate of segmental errors increased after training (36% before vs 52% after; $\chi^2 = 8.76$, $p < .01$), while the rate of suprasegmental errors remained almost constant (9% before vs 7% after). To sum up, for the patients as a group, training of sets of structurally related syllables resulted in significant improvements of the root forms they had been derived from, but not of unrelated control syllables. Figure 1 depicts total numbers of errors for the target and the control syllables for each of the four patients individually.

All patients produced fewer errors on the target syllables after learning. Statistical testing revealed that the difference was significant for RK and LF (binominal test; RK and LF: $p < .01$), MK showed a non-significant trend ($p = .073$), and KH made only very few errors overall. Thus, at least for RK and LF, a clear generalisation effect could be observed on the target syllables. On the control items, an increase of errors was seen in all patients, but was significant only in MK ($p < .05$).

As shown in Table 3, all patients predominantly produced segmental errors. In KH, disfluencies were entirely absent. At a descriptive level, a decrease of segmental errors after the learning trials was found for the target syllables in all patients, which was significant for MK ($p < .05$) and nearly so for LF ($p = .06$). Regarding suprasegmental deviations, both RK and LF improved on the target syllables after learning, whereas MK became slightly less fluent. For the control syllables, a significant effect was only observed for RK, who produced more segmental errors after learning ($p < .05$), but was also more fluent.

---

[4] The slightly lower error rate on the control syllables can be attributed to the improvements in the second session. Whereas in the first session the error rate was nearly the same on the targets (48%) and the controls (46%), there were fewer errors on the control syllables in the second session (targets: 58%, controls: 38%). This might be explainable by a persisting training effect from the first session, where the control syllables of the second session served as targets.

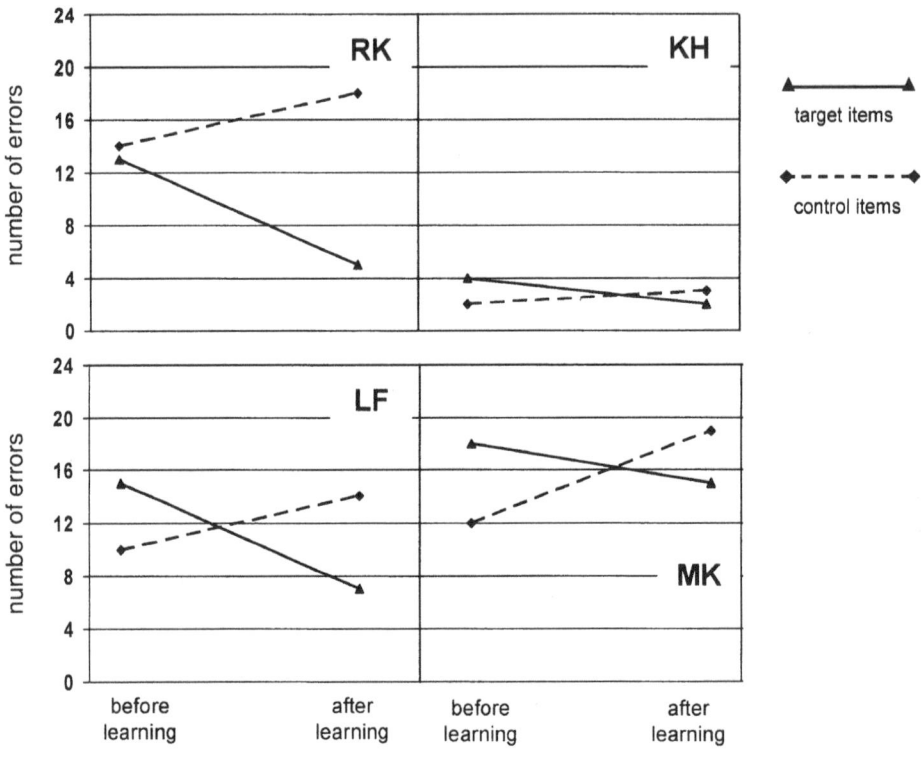

Figure 1. Error numbers before and after learning on target and control items ($N = 24$ in each participant and each condition).

Syllable durations

First, we compared the patients' syllable durations before learning with those obtained from six normal speakers (Figure 2). All patients were significantly slower than the control group—independent-samples t-tests; $t > 4.44$, $p < .001$ for RK, LF, and MK; $t(329) = 2.63$, $p < .01$ for KH. Since the control persons' item durations were inhomogeneous, we also compared each patient with each normal participant. Whereas RK and MK showed a significant slowing in all comparisons ($t > 5.21$, $p < .001$ in each case), LF was slower than four out of six control participants and KH was slower than three. ($t > 3.14$, $p < .01$ in these cases).

TABLE 3
Errors

		RK	KH	LF	MK
Segmental errors	Target	9/4	4/2	12/7	18/10
	Control	7/14	2/3	9/14	15/21
Suprasegmental errors	Target	5/1	...	4/0	1/3
	Control	9/5	--	--	0/2

Total numbers of segmental and suprasegmental errors before/after training, for the target and the control syllables.

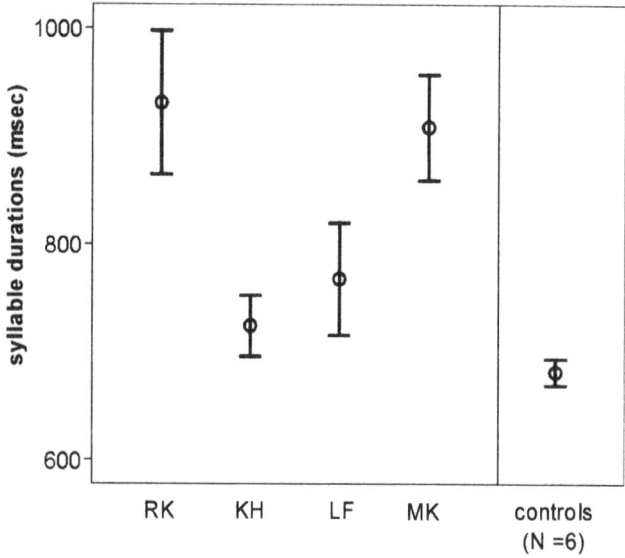

Figure 2. Syllable durations (ms) in the patients (before training) and the control group ($N = 48$ per participant).

To investigate generalisation effects, the patients' syllable durations were compared for the target and the control items before and after the learning trials. In two patients, LF and MK, a relatively high amount of data had to be excluded due to frequent consonant elisions. Because of high numbers of missing values, an analysis of variance could not be conducted. Therefore, separate paired-samples t-tests were carried out for each patient and each of the two stimulus groups.

Before training, none of the patients showed significant differences in durations between the target and the control syllables (independent-samples t-tests; $t < .77$, $p > .05$ in all cases). Regarding changes of syllable durations before vs after learning, distinct patterns could be observed for each patient (see Figure 3).

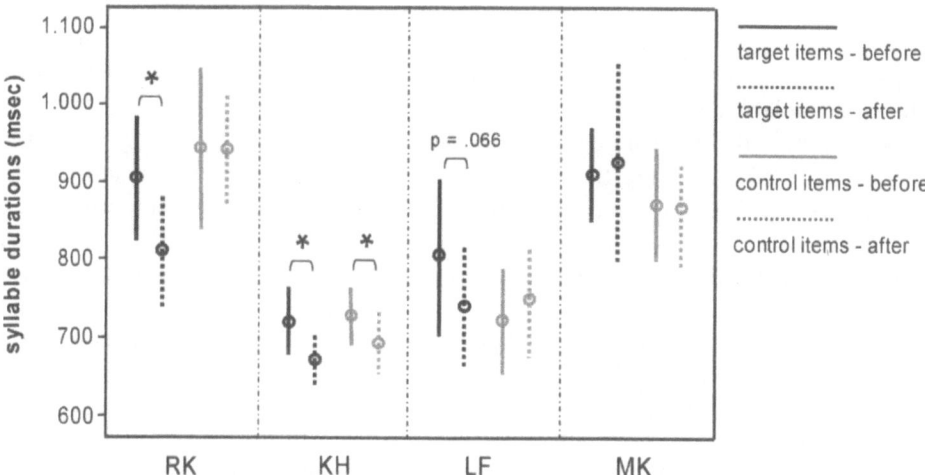

Figure 3. Syllable durations in milliseconds (mean $\pm 2\ SD$) before and after learning of target and control syllables ($N = 24$ for each participant and each condition).

In all patients except MK, target syllable durations were shorter after the training. This effect proved to be significant in RK, paired-samples t-test; $t(19) = 2.91, p < .01$, and KH, $t(20) = 2.5, p < .05$. In LF there was a non-significant trend towards shorter syllable durations after the learning trials, $t(14) = 1.99, p = .066$. In contrast, MK showed no change of syllable durations. Regarding the significant decline of syllable durations in KH, an unspecific effect was observed, since she also produced the control syllables with shorter durations, $t(20) = 2.41, p < .05$. In the other patients there were no changes in the durations of the control items. Therefore RK was the only patient with a specific generalisation effect regarding syllable durations. Furthermore, he was also the only patient who had significantly shorter syllable durations on the target items compared to the control items after training: independent-samples t-test, $t(45) = 2.65, p < .05$.

DISCUSSION

In the present study, four patients with AOS were investigated in a learning experiment. We asked if AOS patients can (re)acquire complex syllabic motor programs by training of different fractions of these syllables. The study was motivated by Levelt et al.'s (1999) assumption that the entries in the syllabary are stored *holistically*. According to this assumption, no generalisation effects should arise, since only practice of a syllable in its complete form would lead to a learning effect of this syllable. On the contrary, if an intensive training of different fractions of a complex target syllable leads to an improvement of the untrained full target syllable, this would be an indication of a more differentiated internal organisation of these stored motor units.

For the patients as a group, a statistically significant reduction of overall error rate and of the rate of segmental errors was observed for the target syllables, but not for the control items. Generalisation effects were significant in three patients. In LF and RK this effect was due to a decline of the segmental and the suprasegmental errors after learning. These two patients also showed specific generalisation effects in their syllable durations. Patient MK achieved a reduction of segmental errors at the expense of reduced fluency. Since the fourth patient, KH, produced only few errors before learning, no significant effects were observed, nonetheless she still showed a slight decline in her rate of segmental errors and, at the same time, became faster on the target syllables.

By contrast, the control items did not benefit from the learning; they were even less accurate after learning than before. This effect, which was significant for the patients as a group, can primarily be attributed to patient RK, but there was such a tendency in the other patients as well. However, regarding syllable durations, RK became more fluent on both the target and the control syllables. The same tendency could be seen in KH, who had shorter syllable durations in both item groups after learning. Therefore, the learning trials may have stimulated these patients to use a faster speaking mode, which they could keep up with for the target but not for the control syllables where fluency was at the expense of accuracy. Another explanation might be that the patients established during each learning block an expectation as to which target item would be trained by the syllable fractions. The presentation of the control syllables may have violated this anticipation and may have caused a problem in adjusting their articulation to the unexpected syllable.

Altogether, in the apraxic speakers examined here, learning of sets of phonologically simple derivatives of complex syllables *generalised* in the sense that the complex target syllables, which had never been exercised, improved significantly after the training. This effect was *specific* to the extent that control syllables, which were segmentally unrelated to the training sets, did not improve.

The specific generalisation effects are incompatible with the postulate of holistic syllable programs that is part of Levelt's model (Levelt et al., 1999). If syllabic motor routines were monolithic entities, only repetitions of always the same syllable in its complete form would contribute to a strengthening of the motor patterns of this specific unit, and no other syllable would profit from this drill. Our findings, on the contrary, suggest that the gestural scores of overlearned syllable routines have an internal architecture and that this architecture can be established through learning its fractions. As a result, structurally related syllables inside the syllabary (i.e., within the motor repertoire of a speaker) may be interconnected and share overlapping elements of their internal make-up. Within such a kind of phonetic network, training of particular syllable programs would also lead to a strengthening of structurally related—i.e., also of more complex—syllable programs.

One might say in opposition that Levelt's theory comprises a spreading activation mechanism from the phonological to the phonetic level and that, on the basis of this mechanism, training of the fractions of a complete target syllable might strengthen the *access* to the complex target syllable (Levelt, 2001; Roelofs, 1997). Under this assumption the observed generalisation effects would not be contradictive to holistically stored syllable programs. However, the signs of apraxic speech cannot be explained as a problem of accessing the syllabary, but are rather indicative of damage to the syllable entries themselves. Therefore, a spreading activation mechanism at the level of syllabic access cannot account for the improvements seen here.

The present study was exclusively based on observations of immediate effects after very short interventions, therefore it cannot be considered as a therapy study. Nonetheless, the results presented here may provide a theoretical framework for future treatment trials. What are the potential consequences of these findings for AOS therapy? A major conclusion is that in syllable-based articulation treatments not only may patients benefit from training effects, but also a generalisation to untreated syllables can be expected as well. Such effects have been described earlier (Wambaugh, West, & Doyle, 1998), but the data reported here may generate more focused hypotheses on how far generalisation effects may go.

If training effects translate from trained syllables to structurally related syllables, one might suggest that a more efficient approach should be based on training of maximally complex syllables, since these syllables have many structural descendants, all of which might profit from the training of only one template. This approach would be the reverse of the one followed here, where many (i.e., 15) simple forms were trained to obtain a generalisation to one root form of overarching complexity. The idea of training complex structures to obtain improvements on less complex ones has already been implemented in treatment studies with agrammatic patients (Ballard & Thompson, 1999; Thompson, Ballard, & Shapiro, 1998) and also in one study with apraxic patients (Maas, Barlow, Robin, & Shapiro, 2002). In our study we decided not to use complex syllables as training stimuli, since we expected the AOS patients to have greater problems with the complex target stimuli to start with and, as a result of their problems, to resort to simplified forms by deleting consonants from clusters. In fact, then, the patients would choose their own way from simple to complex, even if we forced them to work in the reverse order.

Conclusion

In the present study at least three of the four patients with apraxia of speech showed specific generalisation effects from phonologically simple to more complex target syllables.

One of the three patients who demonstrated remarkable generalisation effects had a pure AOS. Therefore, the observed training effects can unambiguously be ascribed to the apraxic impairment.

The data presented here are inconsistent with a holistic architecture of the phonetic syllables as postulated in the speech production model of Levelt et al. (1999). Rather, the syllable programs may be assumed to be representations with an internal organisation. In this view, not only the frequency of the syllables but also their internal structure is a determining factor for the generation of syllable programs (cf. Aichert & Ziegler, 2004; Romani & Galluzzi, 2005; Staiger & Ziegler, 2008 this issue; Ziegler, 2005, 2006). Furthermore, one may speculate that the syllable entries are connected to each other on the basis of their phonetic relatedness. This architecture may be represented as a kind of phonetic network, where phonetically similar syllables may share motor program units at different subsyllabic levels. Within such a model, training of a set of syllables also leads to a strengthening of structurally related syllable programs.

REFERENCES

Aichert, I., Marquardt, C., & Ziegler, W. (2007). *German Database for Sublexical Frequencies.* Unpublished database.

Aichert, I., & Ziegler, W. (2004). Syllable frequency and syllable structure in apraxia of speech. *Brain and Language, 88,* 148–159.

Baayen, R. H., Piepenbrock, R., & Gulikers, L. (1995). *The CELEX lexical database* [CD-ROM]. Philadelphia: Linguistic Data Consortium, University of Pennsylvania.

Ballard, K. J., & Thompson, C. K. (1999). Treatment and generalisation of complex sentence production in agrammatism. *Journal of Speech, Language, and Hearing Research, 42,* 690–707.

Bose, A., Square, P. A., Schlosser, R., & van Lieshout, P. (2001). Effects of PROMPT therapy on speech motor function in a person with aphasia and apraxia of speech. *Aphasiology, 15,* 767–785.

Brendel, B., & Ziegler, W. (2008). Effectiveness of metrical pacing in the treatment of apraxia of speech. *Aphasiology, 22,* 77–102.

Canter, G. J., Trost, J. E., & Burns, M. S. (1985). Contrasting speech patterns in apraxia of speech and phonemic paraphasia. *Brain and Language, 24,* 204–222.

Cholin, J., Levelt, W. J. M., & Schiller, N. O. (2006). Effects of syllable frequency in speech production. *Cognition, 99,* 205–235.

Code, C. (1998). Major review: Models, theories and heuristics in apraxia of speech. *Clinical Linguistics and Phonetics, 12,* 47–65.

Crompton, A. (1982). Syllables and segments in speech production. In A. Cutler (Ed.), *Slips of the tongue and language production* (pp. 109–162). Amsterdam: Mouton Publishers.

Croot, K. (2002). Diagnosis of AOS: Definition and criteria. *Seminars in Speech and Language, 23,* 267–280.

Dabul, B., & Bollier, B. (1976). Therapeutic approaches to apraxia. *Journal of Speech and Hearing Disorders, 41,* 268–276.

De Bleser, R., Cholewa, J., Stadie, N., & Tabatabaie, S. (2004). *LEMO - Lexikon modellorientiert. Einzelfalldiagnostik bei Aphasie, Dyslexie und Dysgraphie*. München: Urban & Fischer.

Freed, D. B., Marshall, R. C., & Frazier, K. E. (1997). Long-term effectiveness of PROMPT treatment in a severly apractic-aphasic speaker. *Aphasiology, 11*, 365–372.

Huber, W., Poeck, K., Weniger, D., & Willmes, K. (1983). *Aachener Apasie Test (AAT)*. Göttingen: Hogrefe.

Levelt, W. J. M. (2001). Spoken word production: A theory of lexical access. *Proceedings of the National Academics of Sciences, 98*, 13464–13471.

Levelt, W. J. M., Roelofs, A., & Meyer, A. S. (1999). A theory of lexical access in speech production. *Behavioral and Brain Sciences, 22*, 1–75.

Levelt, W. J. M., & Wheeldon, L. R. (1994). Do speakers have access to a mental syllabary? *Cognition, 50*, 239–269.

Lindblom, B. (1983). Economy of speech gestures. In P. F. MacNeilage (Ed.), *The production of speech* (pp. 217–245). New York: Springer.

Maas, E., Barlow, J., Robin, D., & Shapiro, L. (2002). Treatment of sound errors in aphasia and apraxia of speech: Effects of phonological complexity. *Aphasiology, 16*, 609–622.

MacNeilage, P. F., Davis, B. L., Kinney, A., & Matyear, C. L. (2000). The motor core of speech: A comparison of serial organization patterns in infants and languages. *Child Development, 71*, 153–163.

McNeil, M. R., Robin, D. A., & Schmidt, R. A. (1997). Apraxia of speech: Definition, differentiation and treatment. In M. R. McNeil (Ed.), *Clinical management of sensorimotor speech disorders* (pp. 311–344). New York: Thieme.

Miller, N. (2000). Changing ideas in apraxia of speech. In I. Papathanasiou (Ed.), *Acquired neurogenic communication disorders* (pp. 173–202). London: Whurr.

Nickels, L., & Howard, D. (2000). When the words won't come: Relating impairments and models of spoken word production. In L. Wheeldon (Ed.), *Aspects of language production* (pp. 115–142). Hove, UK: Psychology Press.

Odell, K. H. (2002). Considerations in target selection in apraxia of speech treatment. *Seminars in Speech and Language, 23*, 309–324.

Odell, K., McNeil, M., Rosenbek, J. C., & Hunter, L. (1990). Perceptual characteristics of consonant production by apraxic speakers. *Journal of Speech and Hearing Disorders, 55*, 345–359.

Roelofs, A. (1997). Syllabification in speech production: Evaluation of WEAVER. *Language and Cognitive Processes, 12*, 657–693.

Romani, C., & Galluzzi, C. (2005). Effects of syllabic complexity in predicting accuracy of repetition and direction of errors in patients with articulatory and phonological difficulties. *Cognitive Neuropsychology, 22*, 817–850.

Staiger, A., & Ziegler, W. (2008). Syllable frequency and syllable structure in the spontaneous speech production of patients with apraxia of speech. *Aphasiology, 22*, 1201–1215.

Thompson, C. K., Ballard, K. J., & Shapiro, L. P. (1998). The role of syntactic complexity in training wh-movement structures in agrammatic aphasia: Optimal order for promoting generalisation. *Journal of the International Neuropsychology Society, 4*, 661–674.

Wambaugh, J. L., West, J. E., & Doyle, P. J. (1998). Treatment for apraxia of speech: Effects of targeting sound groups. *Aphasiology, 12*, 731–743.

Ziegler, W. (2002). Psycholinguistic and motor theories of apraxia of speech. *Seminars in Speech and Language, 23*, 231–243.

Ziegler, W. (2005). A nonlinear model of word length effects in apraxia of speech. *Cognitive Neuropsychology, 22*, 603–623.

Ziegler, W. (2007). Apraxia of speech. In B. Miller & G. Goldenberg (Eds.), *Handbook of clinical neurology*. London: Elsevier.

APHASIOLOGY, 2008, 22 (11), 1230–1247

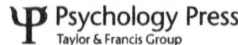

The domain of phonetic encoding in apraxia of speech: Which sub-lexical units count?

Wolfram Ziegler, Anne-Kathrin Thelen, Anja Staiger and Michaela Liepold

City Hospital Bogenhausen, München, Germany

Background: Apraxia of speech (AOS) is generally viewed as a disorder of phonetic encoding. According to current theories, the phonetic encoding process is considered to be based on linear strings of holistic speech motor representations of the size of sublexical units (e.g., phonemes or syllables). This type of model predicts that error rate in apraxia of speech is proportional to the number of phonetic encoding units in an utterance and is not systematically influenced by structural factors originating above or below the level of the critical unit.

Aims: In the present study we tested this prediction for five models based on different units of phonetic encoding.

Methods and Procedures: Ten patients with AOS were examined with a list of words of varying phonological complexity. Phoneme errors in word repetition were counted in different ways, according to five models postulating different domains of phonetic encoding. Linear regression analyses were used to examine the scores obtained for these models for influences of structural factors.

Outcomes & Results: No sublexical unit could be identified that was not systematically influenced by one of the structural factors describing the materials. Major influencing factors were (1) the complexity of syllable constituents and (2) the number of metrical feet in a word.

Conclusions: A model of phonetic encoding in apraxia of speech is proposed that is based on a hierarchy of structural relationships rather than on linearly ordered, holistic programming units. This model may also contain clues for a theory of normal processing mechanisms.

Keywords: Apraxia of speech; Phonemic error; Syllable; Metrical foot; Phonetic encoding.

Apraxia of speech (AOS) is considered as a disorder affecting the process of phonetic encoding in spoken language production. A most important symptom seen in patients with this impairment is that they commit "phonemic" errors, i.e., they omit, substitute, transpose, or add speech segments (Croot, 2002). The term *phonemic* relates to the fact that the units surfacing as the target of the error mechanism are

Address correspondence to: Dr Wolfram Ziegler, EKN – Clinical Neuropsychology Research Group, Dachauerstr. 164, D-80992 München, Germany. E-mail: wolfram.ziegler@extern.lrz-muenchen.de

This study was supported by a grant from the German research foundation (DFG; ZI 469/10-2). We would like to thank ReHa-Hilfe e.V. for additional support. We are also grateful to our colleagues from the Neuropsychological Clinic, Bogenhausen Hospital, München, for their collaboration on clinical issues, and to Katrin Lindner and Patrizia Noël for discussions of phonological issues. Moreover, we would like to express our gratitude to the participants of this study.

http://www.psypress.com/aphasiology　　　　　　　　　　　DOI: 10.1080/02687030701820402

usually of the size of a *phoneme*. Although phonemic errors ("phonemic paraphasias") also occur in nearly all aphasic syndromes, the mechanism underlying phoneme errors in apraxia of speech is not considered as a mechanism operating on abstract linguistic units. On the contrary, the fact that a categorical error is observed on the surface is by no means incompatible with the hypothesis of an apraxic failure of speech motor programming. Such a failure may for instance cause an unintended velar lowering gesture, which would eventually turn a target phoneme [d] into a well-formed [n] and be counted as a phoneme error. Moreover, it is widely acknowledged that for a number of reasons even gradual motor aberrations may, on the surface, have discrete, categorical consequences (Stevens, 1989). According to the proponents of *Articulatory Phonology*, many if not all of the segmental properties of phonological rules and representations can be explained by parametric properties of (abstract) articulatory gestures and their temporal relations (Browman & Goldstein, 1997). Therefore, phonemic errors in perceived apraxic speech should not be prematurely equated with an error mechanism operating on abstract phonemic units. Hence, when we talk here about phoneme errors in apraxia of speech we consider these errors part of the phonetic encoding deficit underlying this syndrome (Code, 1998; Ziegler, 2002b).

This report deals with the grain size of the linguistic units implicated in the phonetic encoding process of apraxic speakers. If phonemic errors are among the sequelae of an impaired phonetic encoding mechanism, a straightforward conclusion might be that phonemes are the core units of phonetic encoding. This was also implicitly suggested by Darley's original definition, according to which apraxia of speech, interferes with the programming of the articulations "for the volitional production of *phonemes*" (Darley, 1969, cited in Wertz, Lapointe, & Rosenbek, 1984, p. 48). A phoneme-based encoding mechanism was also suggested by Varley, Whiteside, and Luff (1999), who claimed that apraxic speakers have lost access to automatic, syllable-based motor routines and are therefore required to use a compensatory "segment-by-segment assembly route" of phonetic encoding.

However, the fact that phonetic encoding failures surface as phoneme-sized errors need not necessarily mean that the cause of such a failure is located at the phoneme level. For instance, when [to'ma:tə] is turned into [to'ba:nə], the phoneme-based model would say that velar movement errors have occurred within the domain of a phonological segment, i.e., in the organisation of the gestural scores for the phonemes [m] and [t]. Yet a syllable-based mechanism may be assumed as well, postulating that the velar gestures in this example are part of a *syllabic* organisation of articulation, hence that the phonetic encoding failure caused errors in the spatial or temporal organisation of the articulatory gestures for the syllables [ma:] and [tə]. This explanation would be compatible with models postulating that the phonetic encoding process is largely based on *syllable*-sized motor representations (cf. Cholin, 2008 this issue) and that the apraxic error mechanism is related to these representations (Aichert & Ziegler, 2004; Aichert & Ziegler, 2008 this issue; Staiger & Ziegler, 2008 this issue). There might still be another explanation of the error mechanism underlying [to'ba:nə], namely that articulation is integrated at the level of metrical feet, hence the motor program for [to'ma:tə] includes a gestural score for the velar movement extending over the trochee ['ma:tə]. In this case, a single programming failure would account for two phoneme errors at the same time. On the whole, the example illustrates that the domain in which the phoneme errors of apraxic speakers arise may also comprise larger, supra-segmental units.

No matter which unit size one assumes, the theories sketched above have in common that they are grounded on the understanding that speech motor programs are holistic primitives that are constituted through motor learning. The syllable [di:], for instance, which—according to CELEX counts (Baayen, Piepenbrock, & Gulikers, 1995)—is the most frequent syllable of German, occurs more than 40,000 times in a million words, and this frequent use of always the same bundle of lingual, labial, mandibular, velar, and laryngeal gestures participating in the production of [di:] is considered to transform the recurring motor pattern into a stable, overlearned movement program, which can then be treated as an indivisible particle by the phonetic encoder. In speaking, such particles are retrieved from procedural memory, one after the other and in a linear order, and their gestural contents are unpacked for articulation. In Levelt's understanding, "a word consisting of n (...) syllables can be phonetically encoded by retrieving n syllable programs from the syllabary" (Levelt, Roelofs, & Meyer, 1999, p. 32). Importantly, in such a theory the motor information that constitutes the basis of our speaking skills is encapsulated in holistic units of a fixed size. As a consequence, merging these units into a smooth stream of speech movements is the business of the motor execution apparatus and no longer a part of the phonetic encoding mechanism proper. Failures of phonetic encoding would affect each encoding unit as a whole, for example by corrupting the stored movement information. Inconsistent, underspecified, or illegible gestural information may then be the source of phonetic or phonemic errors, trial-and-error groping, false starts etc.

This kind of architecture has specific consequences for the occurrence of apraxic speech errors, since it predicts that the number of errors a patient makes on the phonetic encoding units of an utterance is directly proportional to the total number of such units. In a patient with a severe impairment the proportion will be high; in a mildly impaired patient it will be lower. If, for instance, the phonetic encoding unit is the phoneme and a patient's encoder fails on only 10% of all processing steps, this patient will produce a phrase consisting of 80 phonemes with approximately 8 phoneme errors, no matter how these phonemes are distributed over words or syllables. If, as a second example, the relevant unit is the syllable and a patient's severity of impairment is such that she fails on approximately every third encoding step, in a list of 10 three-syllabic words she will make approximately 10 syllable errors, the same as in a list of 15 disyllabic or 30 monosyllabic words. The core assumptions underlying this reasoning are (1) that the phonetic encoding process operates independently on each of a linear sequence of units, and (2) that the patho-mechanism of apraxia of speech interferes with only this process and affects each of the successive encoding steps in a string of such units independently. These assumptions have recently been challenged in an analysis of apraxic speech errors that was based on a non-linear model of phonetic representations (Ziegler, 2005). The results of this study showed that speech motor programs should be considered as hierarchically nested, tree-like, metrical structures rather than as linear sequences of holistic units.

In order to scrutinise the architecture of phonetic encoding units by a different approach, the linearity assumption was taken up again in the investigation reported here. More specifically, we tested the prediction that the number of errors in an utterance is proportional to the total number of relevant units. For this purpose we compared the error scores of apraxic speakers on words of different lengths and different phonological structures, with the rationale that if apraxic errors are bound to holistic units of a certain grain size, the number of errors in a word should not depend on any structural factor except the number of these units.[1] Normalising error numbers by numbers of units should therefore yield error scores that are not systematically influenced by the structural properties of an utterance. This approach was applied to five different error models based on units of different grain sizes. The units were chosen according to conventional theories of metrical phonology (e.g., Goldsmith, 1990), in which words are described as hierarchically organised patterns integrating segments into syllable onsets and rhymes, syllable constituents into syllables, syllables into metrical feet, and metrical feet into words. By this approach we hoped to be able to identify one specific unit with the expected invariance property, which would then be a good candidate for representing the domain of phonetic encoding in apraxia of speech.

ERROR SOURCE MODELS

Our study was based on five different models of where phonemic errors in apraxia of speech may arise.

Phoneme (PHO) model

This model postulates that the source of phonemic errors is the phonological segment, i.e., the *phoneme*. In this view, utterances are considered as strings of phonemes, and every phoneme in an utterance can elicit an error. Hence, the more phonemes there are in an utterance, the more errors may occur, irrespective of how these phonemes are distributed across syllables. As mentioned in the introduction, the PHO model appears intuitively appropriate, since the notion of phonemic errors is strongly suggestive of a segmental error mechanism. This model also implicitly underlies the dual-route explanation of AOS proposed by Varley et al. (1999).

Constituent (ONC) model

This model postulates that the phonetic encoding mechanism operates on syllable constituents, i.e., onsets, nuclei, and codas (ONC).[2] Accordingly, every syllable constituent of a word bears the potential of releasing a phonetic encoding error, irrespective of the number of its segments. This model predicts that syllables with empty onsets (e.g., VC or VCC syllables) and open syllables (e.g., CV or CCV) are less error prone than syllables in which all constituent positions are filled. Analogous to the phoneme model, the linearity assumption implies that the number of constituent errors occurring in an utterance is proportional to the total number of its syllable constituents and not influenced by structural properties otherwise.

---

[1] We are not saying that all units of a particular size are equally vulnerable. Frequency of occurrence or specific motor requirements associated with a unit (e.g., a fricative vs a plosive at the level of phonemes) could for instance be further factor influencing the vulnerability of a unit, but these are properties characterising each unit as a whole rather than its structural relationship with other units. Statistically, a proportional relationship between number of critical segments and number of errors can be expected despite these influences.

[2] A constituent model based on onsets and rhymes was also considered in Thelen (2007). Due to its close relationship with the syllable model, the onset-rhyme model was discarded here.

To our knowledge the ONC model has not explicitly been proposed so far. However, it is compatible with a weak form of the sub-syllabic assembly theory of apraxia of speech, which would postulate that if the mental syllabary can no longer be accessed, speech motor programs for syllables are assembled from syllable constituents (e.g., Varley & Whiteside, 2001). It is also a subject of phonological markedness theories, which would, for instance, predict that CV syllables are less vulnerable than V syllables.

Syllable (SYL) model

This model is based on the assumption that phonetic encoding in apraxia of speech operates on units of syllable size. Hence, every syllable of an utterance can be the source of an error, and the model predicts that, if phonetic encoding goes awry, the number of syllable errors occurring on a given utterance is proportional to its total number of syllables. Since syllables are considered as holistic units in this approach, accuracy is independent of syllable structure. Since the subsequent syllables of an utterance are encoded independently, accuracy should also not be influenced by higher metrical factors such as foot structure. This is the model that comes closest to the mental syllabary theory proposed by Levelt et al. (1999), but it makes no assumptions about possible sub-syllabic repair mechanisms. It is consistent with data showing that AOS errors are sensitive to syllable-related parameters like frequency, but does not account for influences of syllable complexity on apraxic speech errors (Aichert & Ziegler, 2004; Staiger & Ziegler, 2008 this issue).

Metrical foot (MFT) model

In a stress-timed language such as German one might conjecture that the stressed and unstressed syllables forming a metrical foot constitute the core unit of the phonetic encoding process. In this case every time a new metrical foot comes up, the phonetic encoder may fail. The MFT model predicts that the number of foot-related errors in an utterance is directly proportional to its total number of feet, irrespective of the number of syllables or phonemes within a foot. Although we are not aware of any theory based on this assumption, an influence of metrical foot structure upon apraxic speech errors was demonstrated by Ziegler (2005).

Word (WRD) model

At the coarsest level, the word (or phonological word) might theoretically be postulated to be the core unit of phonetic encoding. Under this assumption, every single word an apraxic patient is going to produce bears a certain chance of making an error. Accordingly, the model predicts that the number of errors an apraxic speaker commits in an utterance or in a word list is directly proportional to the total number of words, irrespective of how many phonemes, syllables, or metrical feet these words contain. To our knowledge, no current theory of apraxia of speech is based on such an assumption. On the contrary, there is abounding evidence that word accuracy in apraxia of speech depends on word length factors (cf. Ziegler, 2005).

METHOD

Participants

A total of 10 patients with apraxia of speech (7 f, 3 m; age: 51–76 years, mean 62 years) participated in this study. All patients were right-handed and had suffered infarction of the left middle cerebral artery. Time since onset was between 2 and 41 months.

The Aachener Aphasie Test (Huber, Poeck, Weniger, & Willmes, 1983) revealed that four patients had no or only residual clinical signs of aphasia, three patients had a mild-to-moderate aphasia (unclassified) and three patients had a moderate-to-severe aphasia (one unclassified, one Broca, one global). The clinical records also mentioned the presence of mild dysarthric signs in four patients.

All patients were referred to this project with a clinical diagnosis of apraxia of speech. This diagnosis was based on a clinical assessment of spontaneous speech and of word repetition by experienced speech pathologists. Clinical diagnoses were grounded on the following criteria: (1) the presence of phonemic errors and of phonetic distortions, (2) the inconsistent nature of the errors, occasionally with islands of entirely preserved articulation, (3) disfluent speech, characterised by many initiation problems, false starts, self-corrections, and visible/audible trial-and-error groping.

Only patients with a clear diagnosis of apraxia of speech were included. The severity of apraxic impairment was rated clinically on the basis of the HWL examination (*Hierarchical Word Lists*; Liepold, Ziegler, & Brendel, 2003). In two cases the apraxic impairment was classified as *mild* ($>75\%$ correct), in six cases as *moderate* (25–75% correct), and in two cases as *severe* ($<25\%$ correct). According to clinical records, apraxia of speech was a predominant symptom and the primary target of therapeutic intervention in all patients. In no case was there phonemic jargon or severe impairment of auditory processing. After referral, the clinical diagnoses of all patients were approved by at least two of the authors on the basis of personal examinations and/or video recordings. There was complete agreement between the clinicians' and our own diagnoses. The presence of mild dysarthria in four of the patients was considered to have no influence on the dependent variable reported here, i.e., the occurrence of phonemic errors.

Materials

All participants were administered a word repetition test based on the HWL (Liepold et al., 2003). The list contained 36 real words and 36 structurally matched non-words. With few exceptions all words were uninflected, monomorphemic, concrete nouns—only among the longer words were there a few abstract nouns or compounds. Nonwords were derived from the words by exchanging one or more vowels or, in the longer words, by exchanging several vowels and consonants. In all word–nonword pairs, syllable structure was identical.

The word and nonword lists were balanced across syllabic length (one to four syllables) and complexity of syllable structure—simple (i.e., V, CV, VC, or CVC) vs complex (i.e., containing consonant clusters)—and there was no significant interaction between syllabic length and phoneme density. For a more comprehensive description of the complete HWL materials see Liepold et al. (2003); for statistical details concerning the selection of the words used here see Ziegler (2005).

TABLE 1
Sub-lexical units and structural variables

	кnɛçt	ˈaʊ.gə	ˈka.ka.du	ˈkraŋ.kən.ˈʃvɛs.tər
N phonemes	5	3	6	14
N constituents	3	3	6	12
N syllables	1	2	3	4
N metrical feet[a]	1	1	1[b]	2
Phonemes per constituent (P/C)	1.67	1.00	1.00	1.17
Constituents per syllable (C/S)	3.00	1.50	2.00	3.00
Syllables per foot (S/F)	1.00	2.00	3.00	2.00
Feet per word (F/W)[c]	1.00	1.00	1.00	2.00

Counts of sub-lexical units and computations of the four structural variables used in the regression analyses of this study (four examples from the word list).
[a]Extra-metrical syllables were counted as separate units at the foot level.
[b]Since the metrical pattern of *kakadu* corresponds to a dactyl, this word was counted as a single metrical foot according to the phonological theory underlying this study.
[c]F/W was always equal to the number of metrical feet, since word number was always 1.

For the purpose of this study, the structural complexity of each of the 36 word–nonword pairs was described by the following variables (see Table 1 for examples):

- P/C: the average number of phonemes per syllable constituent.
- C/S: the average number of syllable constituents per syllable.
- S/F: the average number of syllables per metrical foot.
- F/W: the number of feet per word.

Note that these four variables describe phonological complexity in a tree-like, recursive way, starting from the phoneme level (how many phonemes are in a constituent?) and ending up at the word level (how many metrical units are in a word?). However, differing from an earlier, non-linear approach (Ziegler, 2005), the methods used here were strictly linear.

Correlation analyses revealed that the four structural variables were not mutually correlated, with pairwise correlation coefficients (absolute values) lower than 0.26 ($p > .10$ in all pairs). Hence the factors we had selected to describe phonological complexity can be considered independent.

Procedure

All examinations were administered in a silent room and were videotaped (Panasonic NV-GS180; beyerdynamic TG-X-58 external microphone). Videos were stored on the hard disk of a multi-media computer and were analysed using *Pinnacle* video-editing software. Error analyses were based on phonemic transcripts of the target words included in the HWL score-sheets. The examiners[3] scrutinised each videotaped word for the occurrence of phonemic errors and marked in the transcript the type of the error (substitution, deletion, addition) and its location within the word or nonword. Phonetic distortions that did not alter the category of the target phoneme were not considered in the analyses performed here. The major reason why

---

[3] Auditory analyses were performed by A-K. T. ($N = 7$) and by M. L. ($N = 3$).

we selected phoneme errors as the empirical basis of this modelling study was that phoneme errors can more easily be counted and localised to a distinct position in a word than phonetic or supra-segmental errors. In particular, phonetic distortions often include the transitions between two phonemes and can therefore not be allocated unequivocally to a segmental position in a word. As explained in the introduction, we assume here that phonemic errors, like other apraxic error types, result from the phonetic encoding impairment that is considered to constitute the patho-mechanism underlying apraxia of speech.

Error counts

Phonemic errors were counted according to the five different error models described above:

PHO model. All phonemes in a word that were affected by a phoneme substitution or deletion, and all additions of phonemes, were counted and divided by the number of phonemes of the target word. Affricates and ambisyllabic consonants were counted as single phonemes and vocalic /r/ was treated as a consonant (cf. Ziegler, 2005).

ONC model. All syllable constituents (onsets, nuclei, codas) containing a phonemic error (substitution, omission, addition) were counted. No distinction was made between errors affecting only one or more than one consonant of a complex constituent. Ambisyllabic consonants were treated as two constituents, i.e., the coda of the first and the onset of the second syllable. The number of defective constituents was divided by the total number of constituents in a word, not counting empty constituents.

SYL model. All syllables containing a phoneme error were counted, irrespective of how many sub-syllabic units were affected. The number of inaccurate syllables was divided by the total number of syllables in a word.

MFT model. All metrical feet containing a phonemic error were counted, irrespective of how many phonemes, constituents, or syllables were affected. Errors on extrametrical syllables were counted as well, basing on the assumption that a foot-sensitive error mechanism would also be effective on units spared by the metrical parser. Assumptions about metrical parsing were guided by a model of German phonology proposed by Vennemann (1988). According to this theory, all mono- and disyllabic words of the materials examined here were counted as a single metrical unit.[4] Among the three-syllabic words, dactyls were counted as single units, whereas words with penultimate or ultimate stress were considered as two units (a trochee plus anacrusis or a trochee plus an unparsed strong syllable). All four-syllabic words consisted of two feet, either of two trochees or of a dactyl with an unparsed fourth syllable.[5] The number of inaccurate metrical feet was divided by the total number of metrical units in a word.

---

[4] Monosyllabic words were considered as unparsed syllables. All disyllabic words in the materials were trochees.

[5] The metrical theory applied here differs from the model proposed by Janßen and Domahs (2008 this issue).

WRD model. Each word containing a phonemic error was counted as inaccurate, irrespective of how many sub-lexical units were affected. Since only single-word utterances were analysed, the normalisation basis for word errors was 1.

Examples illustrating the different error counts are listed in Table 2.

Listener agreement

Listener agreement was assessed by having an independent transcriber (the first author) re-evaluate the recordings from eight of the ten patients (alphabetically the first eight). From each of these patients, four HWL sublists comprising 12 words and 12 nonwords were selected in such a way that each word from the original list of 96 words was included twice in the re-analysis, spoken by two different patients. Error scores were averaged over patients and over the two corresponding items of a word–nonword pair, resulting in 48 scores. Listener agreement was determined by correlating the scores of the two raters for each of the five variables. Correlations were highly significant in all variables, with the highest coefficient obtained for the WRD score ($r = .97$, $p < .001$, $N = 48$) and the lowest coefficient for the PHO score ($r = .87$, $p < .001$, $N = 48$).

RESULTS

Correlations between error counts across patients

A first question to be answered was whether the different error counts applied here yielded comparable results as regards the characterisation of a patient's severity of

TABLE 2
Error scores according to the different models

	PHO	ONC	SYL	MFT	WRD
[knɛçt] → [knɛst]					
Total no. of units	5	3	1	1	1
No. of affected units	1	1	1	1	1
Error score	0.20	0.33	1.00	1.00	1.00
[toˈmaːtə] → [toˈbaːnə]					
Total no. of units	6	6	3	2	1
No. of affected units	2	2	2	1	1
Error score	0.33	0.33	0.67	0.50	1.00
[pʀɪnˈtʂɛsɪn] → [bɪnˈtʂɛsɪs]					
Total no. of units	9	9	3	2	1
No. of affected units	3	2	2	2	1
Error score	0.33	0.22	0.67	1.00	1.00
[kʀaŋkənʃvɛstər] → [aŋkərʃɛstər]					
Total no. of units	14	12	4	2	1
No. of affected units	4	3	3	2	1
Error score	0.29	0.25	0.75	1.00	1.00

Four original examples from the materials underlying this study.

speech impairment. As an example: Would a patient with a high error score in the WRD model also score similarly high in all other models? In a first analysis, average error scores were calculated for each model and each patient across all items, and pairwise bivariate correlations were computed across patients ($N = 10$). All correlations were highly significant ($r > .97$, $p < .001$ in all cases).

These extremely high correlation coefficients can at least partly be attributed to the fact that the error scores obtained for the different models were logically dependent, since an error score of 0 ($=$ accurate) on a given item in any one model necessarily entailed a score of 0 in all other models. We therefore re-analysed the data by first computing each patient's average word error score (i.e., the proportion of words containing one or more phonemic errors) and then restricting the calculation of all other scores to only the inaccurate words, i.e., to words with a WRD score of 1. By this method we obtained a set of error scores that indicated, for each of the five models, the average "severity" of the errors in a patient.

Figure 1 illustrates the relationship between the scores of the two "most distant" models; the PHO and the WRD models. The two scores still showed a highly significant correlation across patients ($r = .96$, $p < .001$), which demonstrates that patients who made errors on many words also tended to make "severe" errors, i.e., errors on many phonemes in these words. Vice versa, patients who made errors on only a few words also tended to make "mild" errors, i.e., errors involving only few phonemes in these words. At the extremes, the patient who made errors on 96% of all words (marked by an upward arrow in Figure 1) was incorrect on more than 42% of the phonemes of these words, whereas the patient who made errors on only 6% of all words (marked by a downward arrow) was incorrect on only 15% of the phonemes of these words. The correlations between the WRD score and all other error scores were similarly high (ONC: $r = .98$; SYL: $r = .94$; MFT: $r = .88$; $p < .001$ in all cases).

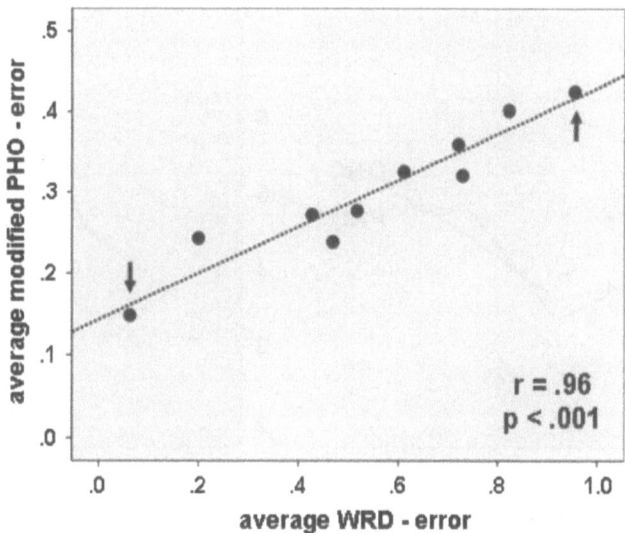

Figure 1. Averaged scores for the word-based (abscissa) and the phoneme-based (ordinate) error counts, for each patient. In the phoneme scores plotted here, only inaccurate words were included (see text). For the two patients marked by arrows see text.

Influences of structural variables

As described in the introduction, the major goal of this study was to identify an error-counting model that characterises a patient's severity of impairment independently of the length and structure of the utterances she/he produces. To this end, the error scores for each model and each item were averaged across all patients. To increase the resolution of the data, the scores of the corresponding words and nonwords (which had identical phonological structures) were pooled as well, resulting in a total of 36 items of different lengths and syllable complexities. For each item, five different error scores were obtained, corresponding to the five error-counting models described above. As an example, the score for the word–nonword pair [te:] (tea) – [tø:] was .25 in the WRD model, which resulted from the fact that five out of ten patients made a phonemic error on either [te:] or [tø:] (5/20). The PHO error obtained for this item was 0.125, which was due to the fact that in each inaccurate word only one of the two phonemes was affected, resulting in an average of 5 out of 40 possible errors. With increasing complexity, the scores of the five error-count models became increasingly diverse. On the whole, each error score provided an index of the "difficulty" of a word within the framework of a specific model and on the basis of the 10 speakers examined here. Under the proportionality assumption, item difficulty should not vary systematically across the 36 items when the appropriate error model is chosen.

Figure 2 illustrates how the scores varied across syllable numbers. It shows, first, that the scores of the different models assumed different overall values: the average proportion of inaccurate phonemes or inaccurate syllable constituents was below .20, inaccurate syllables occurred with a proportion of around one third, and MFT and WRD errors assumed average values of around .45 and .54, respectively.

Beyond these differences in overall range, Figure 2 also illustrates that the five error scores varied across syllable numbers. One-way ANOVAs revealed a significant influence of syllable number for the PHO, the MFT, and the WRD

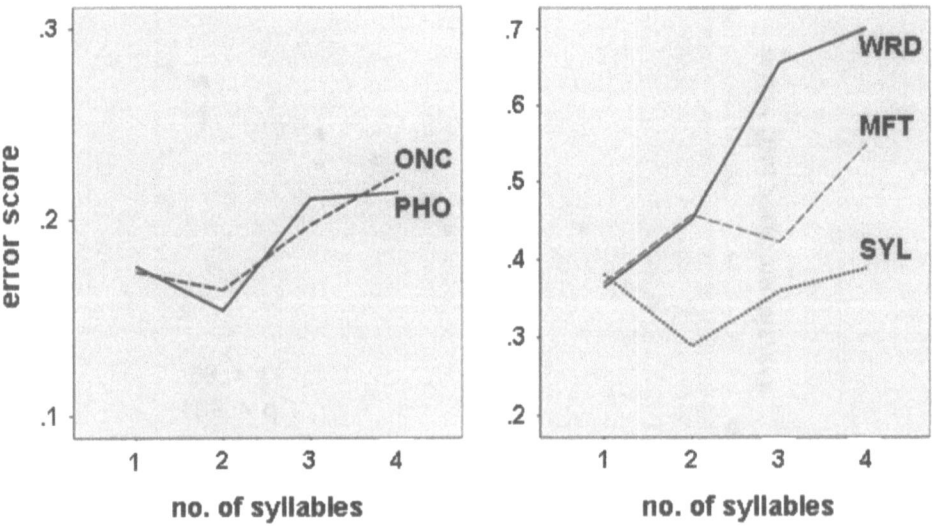

Figure 2. Averaged error scores for the PHO and ONC models (left) and the SYL, MFT, and WRD models (right). The scores are plotted against syllabic lengths of the test words. Note that different scales are used in the two diagrams.

TABLE 3
Stepwise linear regression analyses for the five error models

Entered	PHO		ONC		SYL		MFT		WRD	
	Variable	Cumul. R^2	Variable	Cumul. R^2	Variable	Cumul. R^2	Variable	Cumul. R^2	Variable	Cumul. R^2
1st	F/W	.16	P/C	.13	P/C	.18	S/F	.38	F/W	.47
2nd	–	–	F/W	.29	F/W	.33	P/C	.62	S/F	.60
3rd	–	–	–	–	–	–	–	–	P/C	.75
4th	–	–	–	–	–	–	–	–	C/S	.79
Statistics	$F(1, 35) = 6.3$; $p < .05$		$F(2, 35) = 6.7$; $p < .01$		$F(3, 35) = 5.2$; $p < .01$		$F(2, 35) = 27.2$; $p < .001$		$F(4, 35) = 29.8$; $p < .001$	

Dependent variables: mean errors according to the PHO, ONC, SYL, MFT, or WRD model, respectively. Independent variables: P/C (phonemes per constituent), C/S (constituents per syllable), S/F (syllables per foot), F/W (feet per word). Only significant variables are listed ($p < .05$).

model, $F(3, 35) > 3$, $p < .05$ in all cases, but not for the ONC and the SYL model ($F < 2.3$). Note that in the syllable-wise error counts two-syllabic words were "easier" than monosyllabic words (Figure 2, right), a difference that was significant when only these two word groups were compared by a t-test ($t = 2.2$, $p < .05$).

Syllabic length is only one potentially influencing factor. In order to scrutinise structural influences on the error scores more systematically, the quasi-orthogonal factors listed in Table 1 were used as independent variables in multiple linear regression models, with the five error scores as dependent variables. A method with stepwise inclusion of the predictor variables was used in order to identify the variable(s) influencing the error scores of each model and their relative importance in explaining the variation of error scores across words (probability of F to enter: $p < .05$; probability of F to remove: $p > .10$).

Table 3 reports the results of these regression analyses. In each of the five columns, the variables entering the regression equation for the respective error-counting models are listed in the order of their selection (i.e., of their relative importance in the regression model). The table also contains the corresponding cumulative R^2 values, which increased stepwise with each new variable being entered into the regression model. The maximum R^2 value in each column denotes the overall proportion of the variance explained by the complete model. The bottom line of Table 3 lists the statistics for each model, with the corresponding F-value and the significance level.[6]

Table 3 shows that the amount of variance that could be explained by the four factors was lowest for the finest-grain model (PHO model, $R^2 = .16$) and highest for the coarsest grain model (WRD model, $R^2 = .79$), with a monotonous increase in between. For each of the five models, at least one influencing structural parameter was found.

The PHO scores, to begin with, were modulated significantly by the number of feet in a word, with no other significant predictors in the regression model. This

___
[6] Following a suggestion from one of the reviewers we re-analysed the data by using arcsine-transformed error scores, without finding any difference regarding the results of the multiple linear regression analyses.

influence of metrical complexity can also be inferred from the data plotted in Figure 2 (left), considering that all of the one- and two-syllabic words consisted of a single metrical unit and most of the three-syllabic and all four-syllabic words had two metrical units: the PHO score differences between one- and two-syllabic or three- and four-syllabic words were only small, whereas a larger difference was seen between the two- and the three-syllabic words, i.e., at the boundary between one and two metrical foot units. Hence, in a word with, say, 10 phonemes, 1.6 phoneme errors would occur when the phonemes are distributed over a single metrical foot, whereas 2.1 corrupted phonemes are expected to occur when the word has two metrical units (see Figure 2).

The number of feet remained an influencing factor in all models except the (foot-based) MFT model itself.

As a second important factor, the average number of phonemes per constituent— i.e., the factor P/C—played a significant role in all models above the phoneme level, indicating that the presence of consonant clusters influenced accuracy in all error-counting models except the PHO model. The complexity of metrical feet (i.e., the factor S/F) had a prominent influence on the MFT and the WRD errors, whereas the relative number of constituents was not very influential overall, with a weak influence only on the WRD scores. In the coarsest-grain model, the WRD model, all structural factors were entered in the regression equation, while in the finest-grain model only the number of metrical units was influential. At the intermediate level of the SYL model, influences from lower levels (phonemes per constituent) and from higher levels (feet per word) were found.

One might argue that the metrical influence seen in the PHO model resulted from the fact that this model makes no distinction between vowels and consonants, and that vowels may be less susceptible to apraxic errors than consonants: In words with more than one consonant per syllable, the relative proportion of vocalic segments decreases with increasing syllable number, hence the higher PHO error scores in the words consisting of more than one metrical unit may reflect an influence of consonants rather than of metrical structure. Although this argument would also predict an influence of the number of syllables per foot, which was not observed, we re-calculated the PHO model by normalising phoneme errors relative to the total number of consonants in a word rather than to phoneme number. We also replaced the complexity factor P/C by a factor expressing the number of consonants per syllable constituent, not counting nuclei as constituents. A new regression analysis for the consonant error model now revealed that the error score was no longer influenced by the metrical foot factor. Instead, a significant influence of the number of constituents per syllable was obtained ($R^2 = .31$), $F(1, 35) = 15.2, p < .001$, with a negative coefficient in the regression equation. This indicates that when a given number of consonants are distributed over fewer constituents, the consonant error increases (consonant cluster effect). In order to examine if the influence of the foot factor had entirely disappeared in the consonant model, we additionally compared the error scores of words with one vs two metrical foot units in a t-test. Mean consonant error scores differed significantly between the two groups of words ($t = -2.2, p < .05$). The proportion of corrupted consonants was 29% for words containing one metrical unit and 36% for units containing more than a single foot. On the whole, the metrical effect obviously persisted in the consonant-based PHO model, although it was less prominent.

Homogeneity across severity of impairment

The structural influences seen in the regression analyses documented in Table 3 may at least partly reflect a blend of different patterns depending on differences in the severity of impairment of the 10 patients, rather than a pattern that uniformly characterises all patients. For instance, higher-level effects may have been more important for patients with less severe impairments. In order to test this possibility, a split-half procedure was used to divide the patient group into subgroups of mild and moderate AOS, respectively ($N = 5$ patients each). The error scores for the five different models were re-calculated for each of the two subgroups separately, resulting in two variables for each error score model, one representing mild AOS, the other moderate AOS. Due to a ceiling effect in the mild group, only the two most influencing factors could be tested, i.e., feet per word (F/W) and phonemes per constituent (P/C). For each model, a MANOVA was performed with Severity as a repeated-measures factor and with the two structural variables, F/W and P/C, as between-subjects factors. Since P/C (other than F/W, which was either 1 or 2) was not a categorial variable, the items were grouped into a "low-density" (P/C $\leqslant$ 1) and a "high-density" subgroup (P/C > 1).

The five MANOVAs revealed, as expected, a highly significant main effect of Severity throughout, which was due to the split-half grouping of the patients, $F(1, 32) > 180$, $p < .001$ in all cases. Further, the main effects of the two structural variables confirmed what was already seen in the regression analyses (see Table 3): there was a significant effect of phoneme density (i.e., dichotomised P/C) on all scores except the PHO score ($F > 6.5$, $p < .05$), and a significant effect of foot number on all scores except the MFT score ($F > 5.4$, $p < .05$). Most importantly, however, in none of the models did we find a significant interaction between Severity, on the one hand, and phoneme density or foot number, on the other ($F < 1.9$, $p > .05$ in all five models), which indicates that the error patterns of the two subgroups with mild and moderate apraxia of speech were modulated by the same structural influences.

DISCUSSION

In this study, phonemic errors in word repetition of 10 patients with apraxia of speech were analysed according to five different error unit models. Each of these models was based on the assumption that phonetic encoding in apraxia of speech operates on sub-lexical units of a certain grain size or on whole words, and that the apraxic error mechanism creates errors on these units independent of any structural factors other than the total number of encoding units. The five models differed by their assumptions about the grain size of phonetic encoding units, starting with a phoneme-based model and ending up with a model based on word-sized units. With this approach we tried to sound the limits of linear theories of a phonetic encoding impairment underlying apraxia of speech.

As a first result, the different ways of counting phonemic errors yielded comparable measures of the relative severity of impairment of the 10 patients, since the five error scores were highly correlated with each other. Even when logical dependencies between the different error counts were eliminated, the correlations showed that patients who are likely to make errors on many words of a list are also likely to make errors on many phonemes, constituents, or syllables in a word. This finding, which replicates the results of an earlier study (Ziegler, 2002a, section 3.2.2.3), has an important clinical consequence, since it permits the use of a relatively simple word-based pass–fail evaluation of word production in the assessment of apraxia of speech. As far as only the overall severity of impairment is concerned, no relevant information seems to be lost when phonemic errors are assessed by just counting accurate words, provided that the materials contain a broad variety of "easy" and "difficult" words, as in the Hierarchical Word Lists used in this study (Liepold et al., 2003).

The primary goal of this study was to localise the domain of phonemic errors in apraxia of speech to some level between the phoneme and the word. A principal objection that could be raised at this point is that—according to a widespread conviction—the apraxic error mechanism itself probably interferes at the level of articulatory gestures or of phonetic features rather than at segmental or supra-segmental levels. Hence, what goes wrong in an error such as the one cited in the introduction, where [to'ma:tə] was turned into [to'ba:nə], can most obviously be described as an error at a level where the velar movement distinguishing nasal [m] from oral [b] and oral [t] from nasal [n] interacts with other articulations. Such a mechanism can also account for the many phonetic distortions we observe in apraxia of speech. In this view, a major weakness of the present investigation might have been that levels below the segment were not included at all in the analyses. However, as explained in the introduction, we have to distinguish between the phonetic encoding failure, which presumably operates on some motor integration level above the phoneme, and its consequences at the level of the phonetic integration of sub-segmental, gestural events. Theories of phonetic encoding assume that articulatory gestures are not actually controlled at the level of segment-related or sub-segmental phonetic features, but are integrated into motor programs of a larger grain size and can therefore be controlled from higher representational levels. Therefore, if a velar movement goes awry in an apraxic speaker, the locus of the mechanism releasing this error need not necessarily be ascribable to the instance of this particular movement; a more reasonable assumption is that rather that the organisation of an integrated bundle of gestures extending over some larger domain of phonetic encoding is corrupted. The study reported here was concerned with the question of whether such higher-level integration mechanisms can still be discovered in the speech production of patients who suffer from a deconstruction of the phonetic encoding process, and if they can be located to a particular phonological unit.

The major result of this investigation was that we failed to identify any single unit that satisfied the invariance requirement implicated by the linearity assumption. No matter which unit was postulated as the domain of the phonetic encoding deficit of apraxic speakers, we always found structural variables that systematically influenced the respective error score, meaning that the variance in the occurrence of errors was in no case exhausted simply by the number of units. On the whole, two major influencing factors were seen, i.e., the complexity of syllable structure as expressed by the relative number of phonemes per syllable constituent, and the metrical complexity of words as expressed by the number of metrical units (feet or unparsed syllables) in a word.

Complexity of syllable constituents (the factor P/C), to begin with, had a prominent influence on all error counts above the phoneme level. Hence, when we simply count whether or not a syllable constituent, a syllable, a metrical foot, or a word contains an error, we neglect that the accuracy of these units depends on how many consonants there are in their onsets or their codas. In particular, syllable constituents cannot be considered as indivisible encoding units, entailing that it makes a difference whether one or more than one consonant of a complex onset or coda is involved in an error.

This result was not unexpected, since syllabic complexity has often been shown to modulate the accuracy of apraxic speech (for references see Staiger & Ziegler, 2008 this issue). In the context of this study it demonstrates that units with a grain-size larger than the phoneme cannot be viewed as holistic units of phonetic planning in apraxia of speech. If the syllable is considered to play a prominent role in the apraxic error mechanism (Aichert & Ziegler, 2004; Staiger & Ziegler, 2008 this issue), the syllable complexity effect seen here and elsewhere forces us to assume that the internal architecture of syllable-sized phonetic representations influences the probability of an encoding failure.

Second, our results showed that the number of metrical foot units had an influence on all levels except the metrical foot level. In the model based on phoneme-wise error counts this was the only factor that had a significant influence. After correcting the PHO model for a potential influence of a lower error susceptibility of vowels, the foot effect became smaller but was still detectable in a comparison of mean values of words with one vs two metrical feet. The number of feet in a word was also influential in the models based on syllable constituents (ONC) or on syllables (SYL), which validates the data obtained for the PHO model.

These observations are incompatible with the assumption that the phonetic encoder of apraxic speakers operates solely on sub-syllabic units, as postulated by the two-route account of apraxia of speech (Varley & Whiteside, 2001), since a word's metrical structure is not visible at this level. An explanation for the observed metrical effect might therefore be that phonetic representations include information concerning the foot-structure of an utterance, and that apraxic speakers still have access to this information. A similar result was obtained in an earlier investigation of segmental errors in apraxia of speech (Ziegler, 2005): In this study, error analyses based on a hierarchical, non-linear model of phonetic representations revealed that the concatenation of two syllables had a mitigating affect on accuracy when the two syllables formed a metrical foot, suggesting that the structural unit of metrical feet contributes to an integration of articulatory gestures and may therefore be considered part of the architecture of speech motor programs. In the linear analysis undertaken here, the vulnerability of a word for apraxic failure, no matter how it was measured, showed a supra-additive influence of the number of metrical foot units.

The two remaining structural factors were influential as well, although their influence was less prominent. The number of syllables per foot (S/F), which indicated how complex the metrical feet of a word were, influenced the scores of the two models located above the syllable level, i.e., the MFT and WRD models. As a consequence, counting errors by numbers of corrupted feet or words would neglect that complex feet consisting of two or three syllables are more vulnerable to apraxic failure than metrical units consisting of only one syllable.

The number of constituents per syllable (C/S), which accounted for the presence or absence of syllable onsets and codas, had the smallest effects of all structural factors examined here. It influenced the word-based error-counting model, though only to a minor extent, but especially for the syllable- and foot-based error counts it made no difference how complex the involved syllables were in terms of having an onset and/or a coda. One explanation for this result may be that the materials used here contained only very few words in which syllable *onsets* were lacking. Open syllables (i.e., syllables lacking a coda) were much more frequent, but the presence or absence of a coda may actually have a small effect on accuracy. The findings of Ziegler (2005), for instance, showed that inclusion of a coda position in a rhyme mitigated accuracy relative to what was expected from the inclusion of one or more additional segments, a result that was consistent with the view that the VC link in a syllabic rhyme constitutes a relatively strong cohesive tie (Krakow, 1999). For the data reported here the question remains if a stronger C/S-effect would have been obtained if the materials had been more variable regarding the presence and absence of syllable *onsets*.

On the whole, no single linguistic unit was found here that would explain the occurrence of phonetic encoding failures in apraxia of speech by an approach based on linearly ordered, holistic motor programs. As a consequence, the enterprise of searching for a phonetic encoding unit that is (1) holistic in the sense that its internal architecture has no influence on the phonetic encoding mechanism and (2) independent in the sense that its processing is not influenced by higher-level features was not successful, in the end. A straightforward explanation of this outcome is that phonetic encoding of a word or a phrase involves more than just the retrieval of a sequence of encapsulated programs of a certain grain size. Considering the syllable as theoretically the most plausible candidate of a phonetic programming unit, Levelt et al. (1999) had already conceded that a more elaborate theory of phonetic encoding would "either require larger, word-size stored gestural scores or an additional mechanism of phonetic composition (or both)" (p. 5). The data presented here suggest that the metrical foot could be the domain of such a mechanism. Levelt's theory also stipulates a processing route for the assembly of motor programs from smaller units, although not as the default, but rather as a back-up mechanism when ready-made syllable programs are unavailable (cf. Cholin, 2008 this issue). The importance of smaller bits became apparent in our investigation as well, although in a very distinct sense, i.e., as an influence of the complexity of syllable constituents.

One of the limitations of this study is that our data do not allow us to definitely decide if the different structural factors identified here were influential at the same time in each patient, or if different patients contributed different influencing factors to the overall pattern seen here. However, we were able to exclude the possibility that the different structural effects simply reflected different degrees of severity of apraxic impairment. Hence, our final conclusion is that the domain of phonetic encoding extends over several levels of a hierarchically organised architecture of spoken words and phrases, and that the complex internal structure of phonetic representations is still preserved in patients with apraxia of speech.

REFERENCES

Aichert, I., & Ziegler, W. (2004). Syllable frequency and syllable structure in apraxia of speech. *Brain and Language, 88*, 148–159.

Aichert, I., & Ziegler, W. (2008). Learning a syllable from its parts: Cross-syllabic generalisation effects in patients with apraxia of speech. *Aphasiology, 22*, 1216–1229.

Baayen, R. H., Piepenbrock, R., & Gulikers, L. (1995). *The CELEX lexical database [CD-ROM]*. Linguistic Data Consortium, University of Pennsylvania, PA, Philadelphia.

Browman, C. P., & Goldstein, L. (1997). The gestural phonology model. In W. Hulstijn, H. F. M. Peters, & P. H. H. M. v. Lieshout (Eds.), *Speech production: Motor control, brain research and fluency disorders* (1st ed., pp. 57–71). Amsterdam: Elsevier Science B.V.

Cholin, J. (2008). The mental syllabary in speech production: An integration of different approaches and domains. *Aphasiology, 22*, 1127–1141.

Code, C. (1998). Models, theories and heuristics in apraxia of speech. *Clinical Linguistics and Phonetics, 12*, 47–65.

Croot, K. (2002). Diagnosis of AOS: Definition and criteria. *Seminars in Speech and Language, 23*, 267–280.

Goldsmith, J. A. (1990). *Autosegmental and Metrical Phonology.* Oxford: Basil Blackwell.

Huber, W., Poeck, K., Weniger, D., & Willmes, K. (1983). *Aachener Apasie Test (AAT).* Göttingen: Hogrefe.

Janßen, U., & Domahs, F. (2008). Going on with optimised feet: Evidence for the interaction between segmental and metrical structure in phonological encoding from a case of primary progressive aphasia. *Aphasiology, 22*, 1157–1175.

Krakow, R. A. (1999). Physiological organisation of syllables: A review. *Journal of Phonetics, 27*, 33–54.

Levelt, W. J. M., Roelofs, A., & Meyer, A. S. (1999). A theory of lexical access in speech production. *Behavioral and Brain Sciences, 22*, 1–38.

Liepold, M., Ziegler, W., & Brendel, B. (2003). *Hierarchische Wortlisten. Ein Nachsprechtest für die Sprechapraxiediagnostik.* Dortmund, Borgmann.

Staiger, A., & Ziegler, W. (2008). Syllable frequency and syllable structure in the spontaneous speech production of patients with apraxia of speech. *Aphasiology, 22*, 1201–1215.

Stevens, K. N. (1989). On the quantal nature of speech. *Journal of Phonetics, 17*, 3–45.

Thelen, A.-K. (2007). *Zum Mechanismus der phonematischen Paraphasien bei Sprechapraxie: Ein Vergleich unterschiedlicher Erklärungsansätze.* MA Thesis, Institut für Deutsche Philologie, LMU München.

Varley, R., Whiteside, S., & Luff, H. (1999). Apraxia of speech as a disruption of word-level schemata: Some durational evidence. *Journal of Medical Speech-Language Pathology, 7*, 127–132.

Varley, R., & Whiteside, S. P. (2001). What is the underlying impairment in acquired apraxia of speech? *Aphasiology, 15*, 39–49.

Vennemann, T. (1988). *Preference laws for syllable structure and the explanation of sound change.* Berlin: Mouton.

Wertz, R. T., Lapointe, L. L., & Rosenbek, J. C. (1984). *Apraxia of speech in adults. The disorder and its management.* Orlando, FL: Grune & Stratton.

Ziegler, W. (2005). A nonlinear model of word length effects in apraxia of speech. *Cognitive Neuropsychology, 22*, 603–623.

Ziegler, W. (2002a). Auditive Methoden in der Neurophonetik. *Neurolinguistik, 16*, 5–190.

Ziegler, W. (2002b). Psycholinguistic and motor theories of apraxia of speech. *Seminars in Speech and Language, 23*, 231–243.

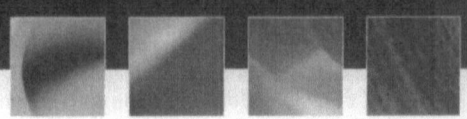
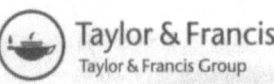 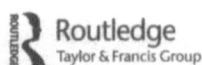 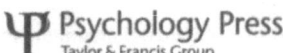
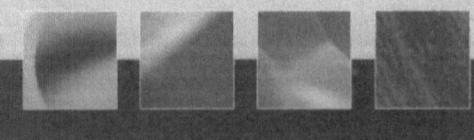